KE
IT O...:

The key to lasting weight loss

HEATHER CAMPBELL

Jean,

Hope you enjoy it,

Heather x

Honeyrock
Books

Published in 2015 by Honeyrock Books

ISBN Paperback: 978-0-9934989-1-6
ebook: 978-0-9934989-0-9

A CIP catalogue copy of this book can be found in the British Library & the National Library of Scotland.

Produced with the help of

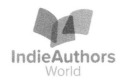

IndieAuthors
World

Acknowledgements

Firstly I would like to thank all the people who have worked through my weight loss plan over the last few years. I hope you have found it helpful. I'd also like to thank those who took the time to read through the first drafts of this book, contributed their thoughts and expertise and helped with my constant market research questions. Your suggestions and encouragements are much appreciated. To the photographer and assistant, I really appreciate your time and patience in getting some great shots.

Thank you most of all to my friends and family who encourage me to push myself and have confidence in my abilities. Without you all, I would never have made it this far.

Finally, the fantastic support, I have received from Indie Authors World and my editor has been invaluable in guiding me through this very steep learning curve. Thank you!

Contents

Preface

Where It All Began

It was the summer of 2009, not long after I'd been to a friend's wedding – where, incidentally, I thought I'd looked pretty good. But as with lots of weight loss stories, it started with the dreaded photograph. And after seeing these wedding photos, I couldn't believe how much weight I'd put on.

In my group of friends and family I'd always been the skinny one, known as the "two suppers girl", for easily being able to munch my way through a fish supper followed by a smoked sausage supper in one sitting – and still stay slim. At work, my colleagues would laugh at the treat drawer in my desk – filled with my favourite crisps, biscuits and chocolate bars. My friends used to laugh and say I must have hollow legs to store it all. With hindsight, it's hardly surprising I ended up the weight I was!

Of course, I'd noticed my clothes getting tighter and my stomach sticking out in a way I didn't like. In fact, if I'm being completely honest, I had been asked a few months previously when I was due by a well-meaning old lady but I seemed to block that from my mind and put it down to an ill-fitting outfit.

Denial is a wonderful tool to keep reality at bay. However, the one thing that jolted me into reality was that photo.

As is often the case, it wasn't just my weight that was out of control. Over the previous few years, the relationship that had never been right for me anyway grew steadily worse, and I'd been stuck in a job that I hated. Nothing life-threatening obviously, but just enough to keep me stuck in a rut and eating for comfort, I guess.

But now something had to change. I credit my therapy training for completely changing my life; not just for giving me the tools to apply to losing weight. And that's the knowledge and experience I hope to pass onto you by writing this book.

A few months before, I'd worked with a client who wanted to lose weight. I'd just finished my training in Cognitive Behavioural Therapy (CBT) and was now a fully qualified therapist, so I decided to do some research into using CBT to help her with her weight issue and ended up using it on myself too!

I'd half-heartedly attempted to lose weight in the past – using some weird soup diet, trying callanetics, paying for a gym membership that I could rarely drag myself out of the house to benefit from. But CBT, and in particular the Beck Diet Solution, written by the renowned therapist Judy Beck, seemed perfect to me as I truly believe it works for many issues, not just being over-weight. And, most importantly, it does not involve giving up any particular food.

I just adore food. Any diet that even hints at the need to cut out a particular food group puts me off immediately, as I do not want my life to be driven by what my diet says I can and cannot eat. If I want to go out for dinner, I will and if I want to meet a friend for coffee and cake, then I do - and I thoroughly enjoy it too!

Luckily, losing weight using CBT allows for all this, and I can honestly say I have never felt restricted in any way by this weight loss plan.

So, every journey begins with a first step and, having re-read the Beck Diet Solution, I merged this with my own knowledge of CBT to come up with something that I can now confirm five years on has definitely worked, and at no point has it felt like a struggle.

You might be thinking that you've heard all this before. I come from a family of self-confessed yo-yo dieters, who have tried everything under the sun. My lasting memory from childhood is each of my parents trying out different diets and failing miserably, having been unable to stick to it long-term so I am familiar with the unreliable results of many diets.

The whole concept of a diet is seen as a short-term thing. People go on a diet until they reach a desired weight, and then stop following it. So it's hardly a surprise that when they stop following the diet, the weight piles on again. It's not rocket science!

I was shocked to read the statistic that although around two-thirds of women and 50% of men in North America and much of Europe are trying to lose weight at any one time, only around 1% of those dieters actually achieve permanent weight loss (Cannon).

The difference with CBT is that it is a series of techniques which people put in place as a new alternative behaviour, for their life-time, not just until they reach a certain weight. Because these techniques are not hugely restrictive or difficult, they can easily be followed indefinitely.

Some of you may be thinking, "Well, isn't it even harder to commit to something for your whole life?" But let's liken it to someone suffering from mild stress or anxiety. Maybe their current way of coping is to go home in the evening and drink a bottle of wine, or always have a sip of "Dutch courage" before going out to a party. If they continue drinking throughout their life it is likely to lead to some health issues, as well as negative effects on their work or home life. A more helpful way of coping with life's stresses would be to practise a short relaxation exercise when they feel their stress level rising, or maybe join a yoga class, or listen to some relaxing music. These techniques would then be practised indefi-nitely to deal with their stress, as they are much more effective at dealing with the problem. Why would they go back to drinking too much if the new techniques were working well?

I hope this book is a helpful companion to you whilst losing weight. My aim is to share both the practical knowledge of how to lose weight alongside my personal journey to show you that it is absolutely achievable. Sometimes weight loss programmes can be a little soulless and – dare I say – boring, so I wanted to bring a real life perspective into what I hope will be an insightful and useful read for you.

Sometimes the very fact of knowing that you are not the only one struggling with a problem can be enough to keep you focussed; so as you read on you can rest assured that I have done and continue to do each of these techniques in order to maintain my current weight. Now, after five years, they have become second nature to me – and you will reach that point too. I keep doing them because they work. No other way of losing weight has ever sustained my interest for that long, and I really hope you find this alternative way of losing weight as helpful to you as I have.

Within this book you will not find ideas for recipes or suggestions for what you should be eating for two reasons:

- Firstly, I am not a dietician. I am a cognitive behavioural therapist, so I am not qualified to tell you what you should and should not eat.

- Secondly, as you read on you will realise that this weight loss plan is not about what you eat anyway. It is about how and why you are eating. It's a whole different approach to weight loss that you may not be used to. That's not to say that you shouldn't try out some healthy recipes if you enjoy them, but there are countless other resources which cater for this so I won't focus on them here.

The main thing I would ask you to keep in mind as you read on is: "It's not what you eat, it's how and why you are eating that's important"

The common theme with all diets is that they promise the earth but very few people can stick to them long term. So I invite you now to read what I did, try it out if you feel you can, and see what happens. Different things work for different people, but what's the harm in trying?

What have you got to lose?

Chapter 1

Common Mental Blocks to Weight Loss

I'd like you to start approaching the battle with your weight from a completely different angle. Firstly, let's replace the word "battle" with the notion that this will be a smooth, simple, achievable process. Imagine practising each step of the way with ease, having the tools you need to overcome all of the usual roadblocks that have previously hindered your journey.

This will involve erasing all that you have learned up to this point and which is currently ingrained in your mind. These mental blocks are preventing you being successful in your weight loss goals and I want to challenge them right now. Bringing them out into the light and being aware of them is the most effective thing you can do to eradicate them, because then at least you know what you are dealing with. I have listed a few common blocks which I have heard others mention regularly, but perhaps you can add a few of your own to the list:

1. I'll wait until I feel really motivated and then I'll exercise

It is a common misconception that motivation magically appears and drives us on to achieve all that we want to. Sometimes it does, but more often than not motivation doesn't kick in until after we have started to make some changes. We are in control of our own motivation levels and can increase these by following some simple steps which we will cover throughout the book. This means that you can take the first step towards a slimmer you now, you don't need to wait until you get a burst of that feeling you have been waiting for. All you need is a little faith that motivation will follow once you get started.

Doesn't it feel good to think that motivation is within your own control? As an incredibly independent "control freak" type of person, I love to think that I am in control over as much as possible in my life. I have what psychologists would call an "internal locus of control"; I believe the solutions in my life start and end with me.

Locus of control is a concept developed by Julian B Rotter in the 1950s, and refers to the extent to which we believe we can control events in our life. Those with an internal locus of control tend to look inward for the cause of various outcomes in their life. They take responsibility for their actions and believe that the outcome is down to their own hard work (or lack of it, depending on the outcome!).

They firmly believe that they are responsible for their own success, whereas someone with an "external locus of control" believes that outside forces, such as fate, luck or other people, determine their outcomes. This can make some people feel a bit helpless when it comes to implementing changes in their life.

If someone believes that their level of success is down to them, then you can see why they would work harder to achieve what they want – they feel it is within their control. But if you feel that some force outside of yourself controls the situation, then why would you try too hard to change it as it would be hopeless anyway?

Everyone is on a continuum of this locus of control. Very few people would be 100% internal or 100% externally focussed. Where do you think you sit on this continuum? Do you think the outcome is determined by you, i.e. "I put on weight because I stopped exercising", or do you feel at the mercy of other people or forces out with your control, i.e. "the supermarket is always tempting me with chocolate treats on offer at the till"?

Being aware of where your "locus of control" lies can help you change your behaviour immensely. If you have an external locus of control then be open to the possibility of looking at things from the other side, and moving along the scale towards the internal locus to help you take control of your weight.

If you agree with the following statements you may well have an external locus of control:

- How can I possibly lose weight when a new takeaway restaurant has opened at the end of my street?

- It's not my fault I'm overweight, everyone gives you such large portions – it's society's fault.

- All my family are overweight, it's in my genes.

Whilst these statements may well have some truth in them, it is not helpful to blame them for your problems. Blame in general is not very productive because it uses up energy that could be better spent focussing on productive behaviours and solutions which lead towards meeting our goals. None of the above statements are very motivating, either. If you assume them to be true, then there is nothing you can do about them so why would you bother trying to make positive changes?

Imagine, on the other hand, that you could look at your situation from a different angle:

- That new restaurant looks good, I'll enjoy a takeaway once in a while, but I'll enjoy looking slimmer and feeling more energetic even more if I refrain from eating from it every week.

- Some places do give such large portions. I know if I finish it all I'll feel uncomfortable and sluggish, so I'll be glad to only eat the amount that suits me.

- Just because my family are overweight doesn't mean I need to follow blindly in their footsteps. I can make changes that will hopefully enable me to reach the best weight I can be.

Do you feel any different reading these statements from the first ones?

If you already have an internal locus of control, these may make perfect sense to you already. If you don't, then they may take a bit of practice to start believing.

Regardless of where you currently stand on the "locus of control" scale, I'd like to think that the second list of statements may be a bit more motivational in terms of allowing you to imagine that you can make a change and lose weight, whereas the first list make it seem impossible, as though it isn't an option.

In short, if you do not feel in charge of yourself or your situation, it is very difficult to motivate yourself to change. It's important to remember in any situation that we do have choice.

I fear I am maybe getting a little too deep so early on in the book, but it's important to be aware of this and believe it. Let me explain.

Victor Frankl was detained in a concentration camp during the First World War – clearly one of the worst situations anyone could find themselves in. His freedom and his family had been taken away from him, which must have been truly terrifying. Most people in such a situation would, understandably, give up and become extremely depressed. But Victor Frankl always held strongly to his one remaining freedom: The freedom to choose how to deal with any given situation.

In his book, **Man's Search for Meaning**, he explained:

"We who lived in concentration camps can remember the men who walked through the huts comforting others, giving away their last piece of bread. They may have been few in number, but they offer sufficient proof that everything can be taken from a man but one thing: the last of human freedoms — to choose one's own attitude in any given set of circumstances — to choose one's own way."

They could not take away his spirit, and he held onto this and continued to do good for others and make the best of the situation throughout his time in the concentration camp.

This is a very extreme example, but I use it to highlight to you that losing weight is a trivial matter in comparison to the hardship that many people face, yet they still remain positive and in control of their own thought process.

You can make the choice now to view losing weight as an impossible uphill struggle, or an achievable target that is completely within your grasp. By choosing the first scenario, you are already on the back foot when making a change, as your mind will be searching for and focussing on all the difficulties rather than the benefits. That way you make things doubly difficult for yourself. Why not choose to shift your focus onto the second scenario for a day, and see if you feel any differently?

If you woke up tomorrow with this magical feeling of motivation, how would your day be different?

```


```

What would you be doing?

```


```

Tomorrow morning when you wake up, do one of the things you have noted here, and the next day, do another. Make a change now – even a small one to get you started – and you will find that elusive motivation is already here.

2. I must be very hard on myself and stick to a rigid diet if it is to work

Actually, the harder you are on yourself, the worse you end up feeling and the less likely you will be to stick to any changes. The more rigid a diet is, the less feasible it is to work in the long term. The key is flexibility and compassion.

The art of self-compassion is a difficult one to master in a society where we are taught to find fault with everything and always strive for more, but if you can be kind to yourself you will have built the most solid foundation for changing your behaviour and, therefore, your weight.

Imagine two small children starting school. One is allocated to a harsh, demanding and punitive teacher who picks out their every mistake, whilst rarely noticing the good the child does. Take a moment to imagine yourself as the child in that situation.

Now, imagine you are the second child who has ended up in a class with a kind, nurturing, supportive teacher. The teacher encourages the child's every step and genuinely praises them for every achievement and even just for trying. She understands that sometimes the child might act a bit naughtily or be distracted, but she knows not to dwell on this. How do you feel being guided by this teacher rather than the first one?

Under which circumstances do you think you would learn and achieve more? Where would you feel most comfortable to try new things and step out of your comfort zone?

Most children, and indeed adults, learn better under a supportive, encouraging influence, not under a terrifying, demanding one. Consider this as you read on. How often do you take on the role of that punitive, demanding school teacher to yourself? Are you ever kind and compassionate to yourself? You might be towards others, but are you kind to yourself?

Many people look at me blankly when I say the words "self-compassion". What is that and how on earth could I be compassionate to myself? The best way I can explain it is that it is the ability to recognise that you are only human, you have flaws, and that's okay. You can't be perfect all the time and, to be honest, why would you want to be?

Practise being kind to yourself every day, even in the face of situations where you have disappointed yourself. Is it such a big deal not to have bothered tidying your house that day, or eating a few biscuits, or getting impatient with your children after a long day at work? Are these things really so bad that you deserve to beat yourself up about it for hours on end.

Being compassionate can be as simple as saying "it wasn't ideal to get impatient but I will practise being more patient from now on" or " I'd rather not have eaten these biscuits but never mind, there are worse things I could do!".

Look at yourself with more understanding. Slow down and breathe. Take a minute each day to notice what you have achieved or to just enjoy the moment you are in, without constantly expecting something of yourself.

There is no special skill involved in doing these things, yet some people find them extremely difficult. Start practising today. Imagine looking down on yourself and smiling, what nice things would you say to a friend in the same position?

3. I can't possibly go out and exercise in bad weather, I must wait until it is dry and exactly the right temperature for me (in Scotland, you'll be waiting a while!)

Why can't you go out in the rain or cold? We are all waterproof. Wrap up warm, wear appropriate shoes, and get on with it. As it is cold or raining for a high percentage of the year in Britain, you are simply putting your life on hold waiting for weather that will not change. The weather is such an easy excuse to use for not going out, but you are really just making it a longer journey to reach your goals.

In an ideal world it would always be a bright sunny day when we are out walking the dog or going for a jog, but we don't live in an ideal world so stop waiting for one to materialise. Just think of the nice hot bath you can take when you get back home, or curling up with a hot water bottle once you have completed your walk, run, or cycle.

If it really is a hurricane/blizzard/flood outside, what's wrong with exercising indoors? Doing something is better than nothing – walk up and down the stairs a few times, go on the Wii, do an exercise DVD, or dance around whilst hoovering. It all counts!

Do you have any other mental blocks when it comes to losing weight? Write them down here and then note down an alternative way of thinking about the situation before you move on:

Mental Block

```
```

Alternative point of view

```
```

Chapter 2

The Technical Bit – What is CBT?

Cognitive Behavioural Therapy (CBT) is the therapy of choice for many common conditions such as depression, addictions, low self-esteem, phobias, and other anxiety disorders such as obsessive compulsive disorder and generalised anxiety. I am a firm believer that different things work for different people, but the reasons why I like CBT are as follows:

It is focussed on the here and now. We can't change our past and we have no idea what the future holds so what's the point in living in either. The here and now is all we have. As the saying goes, "yesterday is history, tomorrow is a mystery..." I find that focussing on this moment right now brings a lot of calm to my mind, because it tends to be our worries about the future or regrets about the past that cause much of our anxiety. Focussing on this moment in time is much more manageable and useful than trying to deal with every possible outcome in the future and regretful situation in the past all at once!

It is goal oriented – If you don't have a specific goal to work on, how can you focus your efforts? Also, I believe people who attend therapy (or use CBT as a self-help tool) do so because they want to change something in their life. Goals help us to identify what we want to change and work towards it. If we don't know where we want to go, how on earth do we set about getting there? This might sound contradictory to the last point, but let me explain.

Although a goal is focussed at some point in the future, the most important aspect of setting a goal is deciding what steps you can take today to move closer to that goal. Dreaming about a distant goal in the future alone is not helpful. You need to take practical steps in the here and now in conjunction with envisaging yourself achieving your goals.

It is measurable, therefore you will know how far along the road you have travelled and if it is working for you or not. I like the idea of CBT because you can see for yourself how it is working for you; there is no big secret within it. There is nothing more motivating than recognising how far you have already come and that you are capable of change, even when you didn't think you were.

It is educational. It puts you, the client, in charge and gives you a toolbox of techniques that you will always have, whenever you meet another blip in the road – and let's face it, that's bound to happen at some point. I also believe it is more beneficial for a client to be in charge of their own life changes rather than relying exclusively on a so-called "expert", which can feel a bit disempowering.

With all this in mind, we can then start to look at how we can change the negative patterns in our life by looking at the basis of CBT, which is the relationship between five important factors:

- the situation or environment we find ourselves in

- thoughts

- behaviour

- emotions

- physical sensations

If we can change one of these factors, it will have an impact on the others. Sometimes we cannot control the situation but we can change our own thoughts or behaviours.

Some people are more in tune with one aspect than another, so we need to build our awareness of each factor. For example, someone very in tune with physical sensations in their body may find it easier to practise relaxation and get their body under control. This will automatically slow things down to deal with negative thoughts or impact on our emotions, by making us feel calmer rather than anxious or scared.

Some people are very tuned into their internal chatter or thoughts that pop into their head, so find it easiest to start by challenging them. This has a knock-on effect on how we then behave and therefore feel.

Look at the 5 factor model below. Can you recognise the pattern in yourself? Practise filling out one of these the next time you feel anxious or upset. The situation doesn't have to be anything to do with eating or your weight, just practise identifying each factor and learning how they relate to each other.

You may start to see patterns in that you always react a certain way, or have similar type thoughts in different situations.

5 Factor Model - Real Life Example

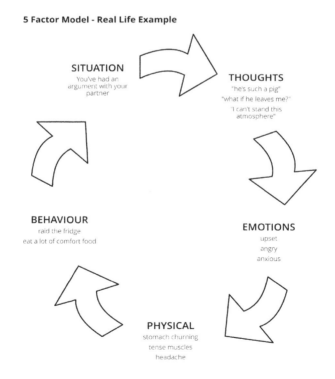

SITUATION
You've had an argument with your partner

THOUGHTS
"he's such a pig"
"what if he leaves me?"
"I can't stand this atmosphere"

BEHAVIOUR
raid the fridge
eat a lot of comfort food

EMOTIONS
upset
angry
anxious

PHYSICAL
stomach churning
tense muscles
headache

Below is a blank 5 factor model for you to use. Whenever you start to feel anxious or upset, or go to eat something you don't want to, plot out the situation on this model to help you identify your thoughts, emotions, physical sensations, and unhelpful behaviours. Not only does writing things down help us make sense of the situation, it also gives us a little bit of space and distance to take the heat out of the moment. This in turn helps us to take positive action, rather than to react in the heat of the moment.

5 Factor Model - Your Turn

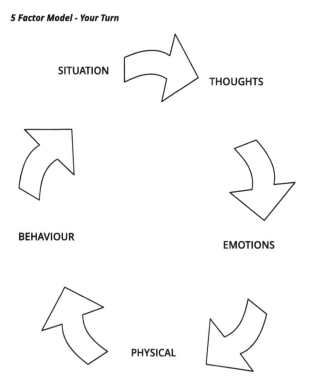

SITUATION

THOUGHTS

BEHAVIOUR

EMOTIONS

PHYSICAL

The focus of this weight loss plan is taking each factor in turn and dealing with it in order to evoke lasting change. People rarely put on weight for only one reason so it makes sense to take a whole situation approach to losing the weight.

CBT is often criticised for being overly optimistic and therefore not taken seriously. In fact, I think it teaches us to be realistic, which may seem too optimistic for a culture that is trained to put themselves down and not allow anyone to climb above themselves. Our brains are set up to find the negatives and look out for the threat in every situation.

Newspapers revel in bad news rather than good, so I guess it does seem at odds with our lifestyle to be realistic rather than completely pessimistic, but that's what CBT aims to do. Think about this for a moment – why is it more beneficial to be overly negative than positive? Surely realism is the ideal mind-set because, as far as I am aware, negativity only serves to keep you stuck in a rut and feeling bad about yourself. Personally, I'd rather have less of that in my life.

CBT was not initially developed as a treatment for weight gain, so you may find that the methods in this book help many other issues in your life simply as a by-product. I have already had this feedback from others who I have worked with on losing weight. They have said it has helped them to feel more in control at work, helped with anxiety-provoking situations such as public speaking, and improved their feelings of wellbeing in general.

This is why I look at this plan as a whole lifestyle change, not just a weight loss tool. Stick with it, it's not as scary as it sounds!

Checklist

1. Focus on the moment

2. Be aware of the five factors interacting in every situation

3. This book will educate you in the techniques of CBT so that you can continue to make these changes long after you finish the book

4. Be realistic, not pessimistic

Chapter 3

Do I Really Want to Lose Weight?

Okay, this might seem like a silly question. Most people will tell you they want to be slimmer, lose a few pounds, or tone up. I don't know about you, but it is all I ever hear about. Losing weight seems to be a universal topic of conversation in workplaces, on nights out, with family, on TV, and in magazines. But if we are all so keen to lose weight, why are obesity levels rising at a terrifying rate?

The first step in the plan is identifying the Pros and Cons of losing weight. The Pros might be easy enough to think of: I'll look better, I'll be healthier, I'll fit into that dress/pair of jeans, etc. But many people's first response to the Cons is: "There aren't any." Well, if there weren't any disadvantages to losing weight, you would be doing it already.

In reality, there are disadvantages to losing weight and you need to acknowledge these and be well aware of them before embarking on the plan. Then you can decide if the Pros, or advantages, really do outweigh the Cons for you, because if you are not completely honest about this, you are starting off on the wrong foot.

For me, the disadvantage of losing weight was that it would involve some amount of effort and a change from the status quo. I also thought I'd no longer be able to eat whatever I wanted. But while it is true that I can't eat continuously without stopping for breath as I wish I could, I haven't had to give up nearly as much as I feared. Quite often the disadvantages are never quite as bad as we fear they will be.

However, maybe losing weight really isn't a priority for you at present. I think we hear so much about it that we almost subconsciously take on this notion that we must lose weight now because everyone says we should be a certain weight or look a certain way, but often it's just not your top priority. Answer the questions below to give yourself a clear picture of the pros and cons of losing weight for you; not what other people or society think you should do.

You will notice I ask the same questions, just in the opposite way. You will often find that different answers spring to mind, based on how the question is worded.

Example:

Advantages of losing weight are:

1. I will look better in all my nice clothes.
2. I will have more energy.
3. I will feel in control of my body.
4. I will be able to buy clothes based on what I like, not what covers my stomach.

Disadvantages of losing weight:

1. It is hard work.
2. I love food so much that I find it hard to stop eating.
3. I hate going to the gym.
4. It means I can't eat whatever I like.

Advantages of staying the same weight:

1. I don't need to change my habits, no-one likes change!
2. It is easier.

Disadvantages of staying the same weight:

1. I won't have achieved this goal for myself.
2. I'll continue to feel flabby and not like the way I look.

Your turn:

Advantages of losing weight:

1.

2.

3.

4.

Disadvantages of losing weight:

1.

2.

3.

4.

Advantages of staying the same weight:

1.

2.

3.

4.

Disadvantages of staying the same weight:

1.

2.

3.

4.

Mull these questions over for a while. The amount of items on each list is not important; it's which points are most pertinent to you that is key. I adore clothes, so it is really important to me to be able to wear whatever I want without jiggly bits of fat falling out of them. So that is a really important point for me, but might not be to other people.

I know, too, that I love food so much that I find it hard to stop eating. Being aware of this means I can work on techniques to deal with this in particular, because I know that all the advantages far outweigh the disadvantages of losing weight for me.

Losing weight should always be a personal choice. Although I feel passionately that maintaining a healthy weight is a good thing for both physical health and emotional wellbeing, and for me it's very important, I accept that for some people it is not their top priority. And societal norms should not be forced upon those who are truly happy at a heavier weight.

If you have made the decision that losing weight is important to you, then it is time to set clear, specific goals that you will visualise every day from now on. I believe this is where many traditional diets fall down, yet for me it is an essential step in setting the foundations of your new lifestyle.

Most people have a vague notion in their head that they want to lose 1/5/10 stone, or they want to reach a certain target weight. But that is not engaging enough, because it is too far away for us to feel like we are having any impact on it. If you didn't have measuring scales, how would you know you had reached this target? How would you feel?

Using your previous Pros and Cons list, I'd like you to write down at least five goals, describing what is important to you, and what you will look forward to feeling or doing when you have lost weight. Refrain from setting an actual target of losing two stone or reaching nine stone, etc, as this plan goes about things a little differently.

Example:

My Goals:

1. I will go out to a party in my gorgeous red dress and it will fit perfectly.

2. I will be able to do an hour's exercise class with ease, rather than feeling like a couch potato.

3. I will receive compliments from friends.

4. I will see a flat stomach and more toned shape when I look in the mirror.

5. I will be able to go into a shop and buy whatever I like without considering my weight.

Your turn:

My Goals:

1.

2.

3.

4.

5.

Now, write these goals on a small piece of paper that will fit into your purse or wallet, write them as a note on your mobile phone, or as a screensaver on your laptop. Stick them up around your house – maybe by your mirror, or inside your wardrobe or biscuit cupboard in the kitchen, so that every time you open it you see these goals.

As well as subconsciously being confronted with them around the house, you need to purposefully read through them at least three times per day. When I say read through them, I mean visualise each one in turn. Close your eyes if it makes it easier, and imagine yourself in that specific outfit you want to fit into, or doing whatever challenge you have set yourself. Where are you, who is with you? Make each one as vivid as possible in your mind; really connect to them.

I suggest setting aside a specific time each day to read these, a time that fits in with your schedule. Think through them in the shower, while you are boiling the kettle, or while waiting on the train to work each day. You will notice that by picking times such as these to read through your goals, it is not actually taking up any extra time in your day – so being too busy is not an excuse!

As well as these specified times, having the goals in your purse or saved on your phone will enable you to read them when you feel your resolve slipping, as they are a clear reminder of why you have committed to this plan. It is so important to constantly remind yourself what life will be like after you have lost the weight, to keep you motivated and focussed on reaching your goals. Sometimes we can get so caught up in the struggle of losing weight that we forget why we are doing it and all the benefits it will bring.

At the beginning of this book I told you that I had seen a photograph of myself at my heaviest and it had spurred me to take action. This is true. I looked at that photo and I didn't like what I saw. That was not how I wanted to come across to other people, and it is not the body I wanted to be stuck with for the rest of my life.

However, as you embark on losing weight it is much more beneficial to look at a picture of when you were slimmer, if you can. Some people may never have been slim so they will need to use the power of their imagination instead. But for those of you who were slimmer at some point in the past, I'd like you to look out a photo of when you felt good, at a size you would like to be.

Even if you don't have a 'slim' photo, it is more effective to visualise yourself where you want to be rather than looking at a photo of your overweight self. Although the overweight photo may scare you initially and jolt you into action, ultimately if you continue looking at it, your mind will be drawn into that state. You will feel bad about yourself, be thinking negatively, and focussing on the struggle to get yourself out of that situation.

Conversely, if you look at the ideal weight photo, you will feel more positive, uplifted, and full of energy to get there as quickly as possible. What we think of most is what we end up doing.

I'd said earlier not to write down a specific amount of weight you want to lose; this is because it is difficult to see the "cause and effect" of your current actions on a large goal. For example, if ultimately you want to lose three stones, it is impossible to envisage how that extra helping of pudding today can impact on that far-off goal. You tell yourself you'll eat the extra pudding now and do something else to make up for this tomorrow.

However, if you focus on smaller increments, it holds you much more accountable for every behaviour. For this reason, I ask you to focus on losing only 5lbs at a time (Beck). Losing 5lbs will be your first goal to reach, and after that another 5lbs, and then another, until you find a comfortable weight. There is no time limit to reaching this 5lbs; it is not a race but a goal you will achieve in time, and much more easily than a far-off, large amount of weight.

When you are aiming for a 5lb loss, suddenly everything you do has more of an impact on this goal. That ten minute walk at lunchtime might make a difference; having a smaller helping at dinner might make a difference. You are holding your actions accountable and feel more involved in the whole process, because you are more tuned into each small change happening and this ultimately culminates in the bigger change.

In order to maintain this level of accountability, I believe it is essential to weigh yourself once a week. I sometimes come across resistance to this at the groups I run, but I think that has a lot to do with denial. It is so easy for weight to creep up and unless you are regularly checking it, it may well be out of control before you realise. Of course you can measure yourself if you like, too, and you should always be aware of how clothes are feeling on you, but I strongly urge you to weigh yourself once a week as well.

And weighing should be no more than once a week, because it's important to be aware of becoming obsessive about your weight, which is the other end of the scale from denial. Neither are helpful to sustaining a long term healthy weight. Weigh in on the same day each week and keep a note of this so you can observe the changes. In the beginning, do this on a weight chart so that you can clearly see any increases and decreases. Something very basic like this would be fine:

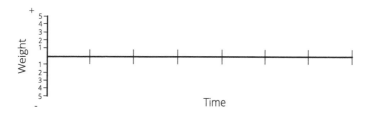

Now that I have lost all the weight I want to and am on the maintaining stage, I note my weight every week in my diary as a way of keeping a record. If you are losing weight alongside a friend or in a group, please be aware that the important thing is to record how much weight is being lost or gained each week, not your actual weight. That means there is never any need to state your weight to anyone if you are not comfortable doing this; you are simply recording how much you are losing or gaining. I am not a fan of group-shaming exercises, as they are counter-intuitive to the basis for this approach, which is compassion and rewards (I'll talk more about this later).

The main reason for weekly weigh-ins, is to counteract any denial and to keep in check with your goals. But there is another benefit to weighing yourself, too. I am trying to foster a realistic approach to weight loss, focussing on rewards rather than punishment.

Every other weight loss approach I have come across has been punitive or depriving in some way. This is not sustainable over the long term. Weighing yourself gives you an opportunity to practise compassion and perspective – two key components in this plan (not to mention in life in general!).

Let me explain. It is impossible to lose weight every single week. By hoping for this, you are being unrealistic from the start and setting yourself up to be disappointed. It is important to keep any weight gains in perspective. You should be looking at the overall pattern of your weigh-ins as declining in general, but being aware that the odd blip in the opposite direction is completely normal. This is a chance for you to practise compassion towards yourself, even in the face of a result you didn't want.

Being able to stand on the scales and see that you have put on a little weight, but being able to move forward from that instantly in a compassionate frame of mind, is integral to this approach. Getting hung up on that little weight gain is a sure fire way to follow the pattern of yo-yo dieting that so many people fall into to. If they put on weight one week, rather than seeing it as a natural flow of weight loss and gain, they view it as a catastrophe. They think, "What's the point?" and "I'll never lose weight", which sends them off on a spiral of overeating. Sound familiar?

Imagine if you stepped off the scales after seeing you have gained a little weight since the previous week, and instantly said, "Okay, I have to gain weight sometimes, but let's get right back on the plan and I'll lose weight again next time." Is that not what you would say to a friend, anyway? Rather than that horrible, harsh, punitive voice you speak to yourself in?

In this way, the scales are no longer an instrument to be feared, but simply used as a tool to keep in check with your goals.

Before moving on, I want to take a moment to explore your goals a little more in depth. So far, you have set goals, but too often people expect diets to be a quick fix and become easily disheartened when they don't get their desired results instantly.

Maintaining weight loss is a big lifestyle change and, as with any lifestyle change, it takes time and effort. Think about other long term goals you have achieved in your life. This could be completing a university degree, or in-work training, passing your driving test, having a baby, saving for a longed-for holiday or your first home. List the goals you have achieved here:

1.

2.

3.

Each of these things took time and, I'd imagine, a good bit of effort. Were they worth the effort? I bet there were times in the middle of each situation that you felt like giving up, or thought you'd never make it – but you did. What can you learn from each of these experiences that you can now use in your long term goal of maintaining weight loss? What skills and characteristics did you draw upon to complete that course or training, raise a child, or save for that holiday or car?

Real Life Example:

When I was studying at university, I was super organised with study timetables, colour co-ordinated notes, etc. This made me feel in control, and I know I work well to a plan. I took these organisational skills and applied them to my weight loss plan.

When I was saving up to pay for a holiday, quite often I would want to go out shopping and buy something nice, but instead I would take a moment and picture myself lying by the pool in a sunny place and remind myself how good I would feel when I was there. So it was worth foregoing the odd shopping spree to get there. Being able to keep in touch with the long term goals over short term gratification is another skill that I was able to put into practice when losing weight.

Your Turn:

List all the skills and your personal qualities and characteristics that helped you to achieve various goals throughout your life. These goals can be big or small.

1.

2.

3.

This is possibly the most important chapter in the whole book, because we have now set the foundations. Setting foundations is often missed out of other weight loss methods but it is absolutely essential. If you build a house with weak foundations, it will fall down; if you start out on a diet with weak foundations, your resolve will quickly crumble, too.

And now you've started. You have set your goals, and are reading through them every day. Well done! See, that wasn't so hard, was it?

Checklist:

1. Be very aware of the disadvantages of losing weight as well as the benefits.

2. Set clear, specific goals for yourself that you can visualise.

3. Think about these goals every day, at least three times.

4. Only focus on losing 5lbs at a time, but do not put a time limit on this. This small amount of weight keeps you accountable.

5. Weigh yourself once a week, and keep a note of the losses and gains your weight chart.

6. Build realistic expectations – it is impossible to lose weight every single week.

7. Be compassionate to yourself, even when things are not going the way you would like.

Chapter 4

Building On Your Solid Foundations

The previous chapter was about setting the scene and building strong foundations from which to work. These foundations are so often missing from other diets, but without them everything else tends to tumble down and fall apart.

Remember from Chapter Two that Cognitive Behavioural Therapy is based on the relationship between our environment, thoughts, behaviour, emotions, and physical sensations in the body. Thoughts are essential to lasting change, and we will look at them in more depth in following chapters, but first I'd like to start you off with some simple behaviour changes which you can implement straight away.

If I asked you to tell me exactly what you ate yesterday, do you think you would remember everything clearly? You might think so, but actually it has been shown that a lot of what we eat goes in completely unnoticed because our full attention is not focussed on it. Many people tend to eat while doing a multitude of other things.

From day one, I found practising the art of mindfulness when eating made such a massive difference to my relationship with food. I am by no means a mindfulness expert, but you will find countless courses and books available on the subject if you would like to research it a bit more. For the purposes of losing weight, though, all you need is a grasp of the basics.

Mindfulness is the practice of paying attention to what is around you, staying in this moment only, and being fully aware of it. That means if you are eating while on the phone or doing the ironing or running around cleaning the house, then your attention is not focussed on what you are eating and you will not register fully what you are taking in. Not only this, but you will not be enjoying the taste of your food nearly as much if you are not focussed on it, so you might feel that you need more to get the same satisfaction.

To start eating mindfully: from now on, I ask that you only ever eat when you are sitting down. There are several reasons for this:

1. It is essential in the practice of eating mindfully.

2. If you need to wait until you are sitting, you provide a natural distraction to cravings, because by the time you have found a seat, the craving has often passed or you have just forgotten about it.

3. By the time you have found a seat and settled down, some time has passed. So you have also managed to stretch out that snack for a lot longer.

Remember, food that we eat on the run is enjoyed less and forgotten quicker. Denial is the enemy in losing weight. Be aware of everything you eat.

For example, when I'm walking home from work each evening, I often get a real urge for some chocolate about halfway through the one hour walk. There are lots of newsagents and takeaway shops surrounding me on my walk home, with lots of tempting sights and smells. My first reaction in the past would have been to go and buy a treat and wolf it down as I carried on walking. Now, I tell myself I can have a treat when I reach the train station and am sitting in my seat on my journey home. I aim to wait and buy the treat when I reach the station, and by that stage nine times out of ten the craving has actually passed and I'm content to wait until I get home to make my dinner.

Sometimes I do buy the treat and eat it and that is okay, because I'm no longer doing it every day, or every time I have a craving. Imagine reducing how often you respond to your cravings by even 50% – that's a huge amount of calories saved.

This delaying tactic is much more effective than not allowing myself any treats at all. Not only is it sticking to the mindfulness principle, which is key to this approach, but a recent study by Dr Nicole Mead has also found people who postponed eating their favourite snack as opposed to saying "no" completely, were able to resist temptation better than those who try to totally refrain.

Dr Mead explains that "Postponement weakens desire at the precise time when it overwhelms willpower". In other words, it is much more achievable to say that we will still eat what we want, only a little bit later, than shout at ourselves and say that we can't have it ever again. It's a simple little trick that your brain will fall for, because cravings only usually last for a few minutes and then they pass naturally on their own. By that time, your brain has moved on to focus on something else.

Once you get into the habit of sitting down to eat – even if it's just for a quick bite of your favourite chocolate bar – you then need to focus on the technique of mindfulness. The aim is to make each piece of food last as long as you possibly can, as the longer it lasts the less you will eat, simply because instead of going back for seconds, you are still on the first! Let's say you've been given a box of chocolates, which would normally be devoured shortly after opening. By eating mindfully, I can still enjoy the chocolates now and again, but not only will they last much longer, they will taste a whole lot better, too.

Open the box and really look at each chocolate. Consider carefully which one you would love to eat the most. What is your favourite flavour? What does it look like? What shape is the chocolate? Is it dark, white, milk chocolate? Is there a flavoured centre? Before placing it in your mouth, smell it; engage every sense in eating.

Now, slowly take a bite – just a small bite, remember. What does it feel like in your mouth? Is it hard on the outside, leading to a soft centre? Or is it the same texture the whole way through? Feel it melting on your tongue. What do you taste first? Is it bitter or sweet? Really slow down and take a moment to focus on the flavours in your mouth. Isn't that delicious?

Even after you have swallowed that bite, savour it. I'm sure you can still taste it in your mouth, and the best bit is that you still have more of that same chocolate left to eat; it hasn't all disappeared in a couple of seconds. Savour that first bite for as long as you can, and wait as long as possible before taking another bite.

How many bites can you get out of this one chocolate? If it usually takes you ten seconds to eat a small chocolate, can you make it last ten minutes? Challenge yourself, because imagine how many chocolates you could normally eat in ten minutes before you started eating mindfully. If you are now only eating one in that same time slot, you have significantly reduced how much you are eating, yet you are still allowing yourself the same treat.

I now feel really cheated if I have prepared a meal or am eating in a restaurant and for some reason have to eat the meal really quickly, because I always feel that I haven't really tasted it and enjoyed it fully. Try this with your meals at home. Time how long it takes you to eat your meal as usual, then on following nights for the rest of the week try and increase that time – even just by two minutes each night – until you slow down by as much as you possibly can.

You may wonder how on earth some of these techniques are going to help you to lose weight, but all I can ask is that you have a little faith in them and be prepared to experiment with new things. Diets you've tried in the past haven't worked, so where's the harm in trying a different way?

When we eat whilst doing other things, our full attention is not on the food, therefore it's easy to forget the snacks we've had through the day. This method is also a way of finding out if what you want to eat is actual hunger or just a craving, as if you insist on waiting until you sit down, you might sometimes find you are no longer hungry.

If we were to stop here, and these were the only two techniques you were to do, I am certain you would reduce your calorie intake. But there are so many more tools that can make weight loss even easier.

The mind-set you adopt to approach this plan is so important to how long you will stick with it. Most weight loss plans are punitive, strict, and inflexible. We know that rewarding good behaviour works better than punishing bad behaviour. If you have children or work with them, you will know this to be true. Children tend to rebel against punishment, and it's exactly the same with adults.

It's also important to bear in mind that whatever you give attention to, it grows. So if you focus on all the bad things going on in your life, you tend to feel worse; if you focus on what you are grateful for, or all the positives through the day, you will feel your mood improving because you are giving more attention to the good bits.

In terms of losing weight then, rather than obsess over less than perfect behaviour, I would like you to focus only on what you are doing well and reward this positive behaviour. I am not advocating that you bury your head in the sand, but it's not useful and can be detrimental to constantly punish yourself for small misdemeanours.

Try and act towards yourself the same way that you would treat a good friend. Would you shout at them for eating a biscuit, or try and enforce a starvation rule on them for the rest of the day because they dared eat a dessert when you were out for lunch? I'd imagine that you would be much kinder and maybe say, "Well, it's done now, so let's move on because I know you can do it" or "Well, you did eat that biscuit but you also went out for a long walk yesterday/went swimming, so keep that up".

Rewards could be 50p in a jar every time you walk to the shops instead of driving, or a long bubble bath if you have managed not to give into cravings that day. A larger reward should be set aside for when you reach your 5lb target. Maybe there is a pair of shoes you'd love to buy, or a pair of earrings, or a trip to the cinema with a friend.

Rewards don't have to be expensive; make them suit your budget or even think up some free ones. A soak in the bath doesn't cost anything or if you have children, maybe arranging a couple of hours for your partner or a friend to take them to give you some "me time" with your favourite book. Having these things to look forward to acts as much-needed encouragement when the going gets tough.

Real Life Example

I was out shopping one day with a friend of mine who was following this plan. She noticed that a gorgeous red handbag she had wanted for ages was in a sale. Worried she would miss out, she bought it – but promptly handed it over to me for safekeeping, with the strict instruction that I was not to give it back to her until she reached her next 5lb target. It worked as a great incentive for her to get there, because she could visualise the actual reward waiting for her.

Rewarding yourself may seem strange at first, if you are not used to being kind to yourself, but remember to treat it like an experiment until it starts to feel natural.

With these new techniques, it can be helpful to have someone to share the journey with. They don't necessarily need to be losing weight, too, but it's helpful to have a friend that you can go to in times of celebration and when times are harder. Take some time now to think who you could share your progress with. They should be completely supportive, trustworthy, and honest, so that they can challenge you in a supportive manner when necessary.

It's a good idea to explain these techniques to them so that they know it's not like a regular diet. You will contact this person at least once a week to advise them of your weigh-in results (your actual weight is not necessary, just what you have gained or lost), but you can also contact them in-between times to let them know if you achieved something like going to a fitness class, or at times when you are really struggling with cravings and need a pep talk.

The contact can be as little as a quick email or text message, but it's good to know there is someone to support and encourage you when you need it.

Real Life Example

It has been several years now since my mum started this plan, but every Thursday morning she still texts me after her weigh-in. She finds this keeps her focussed, and hopefully I can offer some reminders of what to do in the week ahead to keep her on target.

The next behavioural technique is meal planning. Some people find the idea of planning really helpful to keep them on track, while others find it too restrictive. I suggest you try it for a week or so and see how it works out for you.

Creating a meal plan means that you always know when your next meal or snack is coming. In my case, it's more manageable to know that I'll be eating again in two hours as I can look forward to it and fill my time, knowing that the next snack is just around the corner. It also counteracts denial, as what you have eaten is written down in front of you. Finally it shows patterns in your eating habits, so you can identify when you are eating more to try and use this information to balance things out a little.

Please don't take the idea of meal planning too strictly. It can be as flexible as writing it the night before if this suits you, as I know every day can be different. The aim is to allow you to prepare for your day without being caught off-guard with no food.

If you know you are going to be out and about all day, it could be helpful to pop a healthy snack in your bag so you are not caught out and unprepared. Also I find it helpful to make my own lunch to take to work each day. Not only does this save a lot of money, but I know I will have a healthier choice than if I need to buy something in a rush from the local greasy spoon café.

You may also feel like having something different for dinner than what you wrote down in your plan the day before. That's okay. This is just a template which can be adjusted as you go along. It just gives you the chance to plan in healthier choices rather than being caught off-guard and going for the quickest – usually more fattening alternative.

To complete your meal plan, write out a list of exactly what you plan to eat tomorrow and at what time. The key is to eat little and often, to keep your metabolism up and prevent your body storing fat. As Geoffrey Cannon reminds us, "Pig breeders have known for 2500 years that the most effective way of fattening an animal is first to starve it", so why do we continue to go against basic biology by starving ourselves in the hope that it leads to weight loss? It doesn't!

Add this meal planning exercise into your activity schedule (which we'll talk about shortly), to ensure it gets done. It only takes five minutes.

The next day, when you are actually eating through your meal plan, put a tick next to the items you ate. If you were not hungry at that point but ate them later, write down the time you actually ate them. If you did not eat them at all, put a cross next to them and add in anything you ate in addition to what was on the plan and the time you ate it.

This is not about counting calories. It is about being aware of exactly what you are eating so that you can come up with a strategy for times when you feel particularly hungry, and also so that you always have planned food to hand throughout the day, rather than reaching for the most convenient, unhealthy option if you are caught unawares.

SAMPLE MEAL PLAN

TIME	FOOD	OUTCOME
8am	boiled egg & 1 slice of toast	✓
11am	yoghurt	✓ 11.15am
1pm	1 chicken salad roll	✓
2.30pm	1 chicken salad roll	✓
4.30pm	1 biscuit	✗
6pm	pasta in a tomato sauce with grilled pepper	✓ 5.45pm
EXTRAS		
9pm	2 biscuits	+

Please note that this is not a suggestion of what you should eat. It is simply suggesting a way to lay out your daily meal plan.

To finish this chapter, I'd like to move away from the behavioural box of the 5 factor model and turn our attention to the environment or situation. We are very lucky that with weight issues we can at times have an element of control over this box; there are other life circumstances when we don't always have control over this factor. Of course, there will be times when we cannot control the environment in which we find ourselves. For example, my office often resembles a sweet shop with the amount of delicious treats that people bring in for staff.

I can't change this so I have to find ways to deal with it, but there are other situations that I do have control over – like, in my own home. The following techniques can be put into practise in those situations which we do have control over.

As I said at the beginning, I do not believe in cutting out certain food groups from your diet because as soon as you tell yourself you can't have something, it's the first thing you want. So the message I want to get across is that you can eat anything you want, but always in moderation.

This is where we turn our attention to portion control. Again, as with other techniques, I like to take a flexible approach here as I think that is more sustainable. So I wouldn't suggest weighing out ingredients at all.

What I suggest you do is to start by serving up your usual helping of your evening meal, look at it on the plate and then put half of it back in the pot. Eat this smaller amount slowly and mindfully, as described in the previous chapter, and then wait twenty minutes or so and see how you feel. If you are still hungry at that point, by all means go and eat a bit more.

This will hopefully give you a better idea of how much you actually need to feel satisfied. I often hear of people, usually women, giving themselves the same portion size as their husband who is 6ft 4 and doing a physically demanding job, or the same as her growing teenage son. Yet she simply does not need to consume as much as them, and if she continues to do so she will end up the same size or heavier than them.

The aim at the end of a meal is to feel satisfied, not stuffed and uncomfortable. Controlling portion size will allow you to eat the remainder the next night, have it for lunch tomorrow, or freeze it for another day. It's a great way of saving money, too.

Portion control is essential if we are to enjoy a little bit of what we fancy now and again, so start becoming aware of how much you are eating today.

Another way to change our environment is to control the amount of environmental temptations that we have access to.

Real Life Example:

I adore crisps. They are my favourite treat and I would eat them every day (several times a day!) if I could. When I was overweight, I used to buy the big boxes of crisps from the cash and carry which would then be lying around my house. So I would always reach for them whenever I was bored or had a slight craving for them, or just couldn't be bothered making anything else to eat.

By having these in the house I was just making it even more difficult for myself to reach my goals, because I was putting temptation in front of me to tease me at times when my willpower was at a low ebb.

I still enjoy crisps quite regularly but I no longer buy them to keep in the house. I enjoy a packet when I am out, maybe after lunch at work, or I'll enjoy some if I'm at a party and they are there. But by not having them in the house, I have automatically cut out a lot of unnecessary eating without feeling deprived.

It's important to know your weaknesses and remove them where possible so that they are truly only enjoyed as a treat, not as an everyday staple of your diet.

I believe every food choice starts at the supermarket, so this is where you must be most aware. If you buy it, you are most likely going to eat it. Why are you even walking down the biscuit aisle if you don't intend to buy any?

Go shopping with a list and avoid the aisles with your favourite treats. This is where the meal planning exercise discussed earlier can really help, as you can write your shopping list based on what you plan to eat through the week, including healthier snacks.

You'll have heard this one a million times before, but NEVER go shopping when you are hungry. It really does add lots of unnecessary calories into your shopping trolley because it is so much harder to resist these treats when we are hungry.

People often complain to me that they must have unhealthy snacks in the house for their children/partner/visitors. Of course you cannot force your new eating habits onto the whole household, but I would question why you can't buy some healthier treats for your children, too. Surely that would be is a good thing.

When I have visitors coming round, I buy biscuits that I don't like so that I am not tempted to eat them myself. Why would I buy my favourite biscuits when they are not supposed to be for me anyway?

Checklist

1. Be mindful of what you are eating.

2. Always sit down when eating, even for just a bite.

3. Postpone, don't deny yourself food.

4. Focus on what you have done well and reward yourself.

5. Include a supportive friend in your weight loss journey.

6. Plan your food intake in advance so you are never caught short and hungry.

7. Over-eating starts with the decisions you make at the supermarket.

8. Reduce your portion size.

Chapter 5

Exercise

The sole focus of many popular diets is food consumption, whether that is a low fat or low carb diet, or separating food into "good" and "bad" categories in some other way. However, food is only half the story, just as a weight loss plan without exercise is also only half the story.

Many people shudder at the word "exercise", maybe from long lost memories of PE at school with a draconian teacher standing with a whistle while you were made to run up hills in the pouring rain, or in my case play rugby in a mixed-sex team when I was five foot with no muscle up against a team full of teenage boys! Other people have scary images of spending all their free time slogging away at the gym, sweating and exhausted, surrounded by tiny gym bunnies who don't have a hair out of place. If this is where your thoughts take you then we need to re-frame the word exercise for you.

I want you to strip the idea right back and let's only aim for what is achievable for you at this moment in time. If you are currently a couch potato who does no exercise whatsoever, then a ten minute walk to the end of your street is a good goal for you. Or if that is too much, let's start walking up and down your stairs at home once today, then twice tomorrow, and so on.

Exercise is a key component of this plan for several reasons. Firstly, exercise burns calories quicker because it turns fat into muscle and muscle burns more calories. Therefore, having a higher proportion of muscle to fat simply means you will be a lean, mean, calorie-burning machine even when you are at rest.

It is important to remember, however, that muscle is also heavier than fat so while your body is transforming into a higher ratio of muscle to fat, you may notice a little weight gain at times. This is natural, and an excellent opportunity to practise the self-compassion on the scales that we talked about earlier. Remember, this weight loss is for the long term, so a slight increase in weight now is worth it for more sustained weight loss over time.

In Geoffrey Cannon's excellent book, Dieting Makes You Fat, psychologist Dr Traci Mann is quoted as saying that "regular, sustained physical activity controls body weight and fat, not dieting". This is an important message I'd like you to remember.

Secondly, the more exercise you do, the more calories you burn. It is a simple equation, much like fuel burning in a car. The fuel doesn't burn away if the car doesn't drive anywhere. Our body does burn a certain number of calories just to keep us alive even when we are at rest, but to burn the excess calories that we take in, we need to do something to burn them away!

Thirdly, I believe exercise is so good for all round wellbeing. I recommend exercise to clients in some form or another, regardless of the issue they come to me with – whether weight loss, depression, or anxiety. Exercise boosts your mood. It puts you in a more positive mind-set, making your goals seem more achievable. I always find that a problem never seems quite so bad after a brisk walk in the fresh air; much better than sitting stewing over it at home.

There is no point in setting wild goals of going to the gym every night for the rest of your life or running a marathon if you hate the gym and running a marathon brings you out in a cold sweat rather than a rush of adrenaline. You will only stick to an exercise plan that you enjoy and which fits in with your lifestyle.

So, firstly, make a list of any exercise that you currently enjoy, used to enjoy, or have always wanted to try:

1.

2.

3.

4.

5.

My list included walking, Pilates, and some form of dancing or exercise to music. I've always enjoyed walking, and fancied trying out Pilates to see what it was like. I have no sense of co-ordination or balance, but the idea of dancing around to music sounded quite enjoyable to me, as long as it wasn't a serious dance class. I only wanted to burn calories, not turn professional. Zumba, therefore, was perfect, although interestingly I had already lost all the weight I wanted to when I started going to a Zumba class. I joined one because I found I so enjoyed the feeling I got after exercising and wanted to add a bit more to my walking routine.

This is what I mean by long term weight loss. I haven't stopped exercising just because I've reached my target weight. In fact, the more weight I lost, the more energy I had and the more exercise I wanted to do. It's simply common sense that if you stop exercising, then of course your weight will creep up again. But by doing exercise you enjoy, it doesn't feel like a chore that you can't wait to finish.

As a first step, the easiest thing for me to do was to increase the amount I walked. I get the train to and from work, and when I made the decision to lose weight I decided I would replace the second leg of my journey – involving two Underground stops – with a brisk walk to work instead. I had never done this before and estimated it would take around thirty minutes. In fact I now have it down to twenty-two minutes, and I have to say I find it invigorating.

Once I got into the routine of doing this for a few weeks, I wanted to push myself further. I work in two different offices, and the other office is around a three mile walk from the train station in the city centre. On the first day that I had the notion to push myself, I never thought for a minute that I would walk the whole three miles. But I told myself I would walk to the first Underground station and see how I felt.

I reached that in just over twenty minutes and felt fine, so decided to continue on to the next one, a further ten minutes away. I had every intention of stopping at that point and hopping on the Underground, but at that point I still felt okay. So I thought to myself, wouldn't it be amazing if I could actually walk the whole way into the city centre from my work? I was already halfway there so I kept going.

I have to admit, I felt pretty knackered. I could feel the blood pumping in my legs and was sweating profusely (or "glowing", as my very lady-like friend always corrects me!) by the time I reached the train station. It had taken me just over an hour, but I felt amazing having achieved that.

Now, I know there are people out there running marathons and completing triathlons and climbing mountains who would scoff at my little three mile walk, but it is all relative. That walk was something I had not thought I was capable of at that time, and there are many other people who would feel like that is too big a mountain to climb in their situation.

Take note, though, how I built myself up, slowly testing out what I could do. At each stage, I told myself there was a train station or bus stop nearby that I could hop on if I was too tired. This also works wonders in tricking your brain into thinking you are only going to do a little tiny bit of exercise, as I doubt I would have even set out on that first walk if I'd told myself that I was walking the whole three miles.

Setting up too big a goal can be too daunting and we therefore don't even try it. That's why small steps are the way to go. From that first walk home from work, this is now my daily routine. I walk the three miles to the train station most days because I find that it has many benefits and suits my lifestyle perfectly. It is an excellent way to clear my head after a day at work, so that by the time I get home, I have processed the whole day and don't think about work.

I find that exercise really does put me in a more positive frame of mind, and any problems I'm worrying about are quickly put into perspective by pounding the streets. I know that I find it near impossible to drag myself back out to the gym or even just for a walk after I've already got inside my house, but doing my exercise on the way home means I don't have to.

I view this time spent walking home as part of my commute from work, and allow for this time when making plans in the evening. For example, I only agree to meet people after 6pm, not 5pm, to leave me time for my walk home. People so often say to me, "How can you be bothered? It's raining outside/so cold/aren't you tired after work?" Well, my answer to that is – I'm waterproof; I won't drown in the rain; take a good umbrella and you won't even feel it; dress appropriately in a warm coat and waterproof shoes and it makes no difference.

Sometimes I admit that I am really tired after a day's work and I can see the walk far enough. It would be so much easier to get the train at the nearer station and sit and read my book. But each time I force myself to do the walk, I end up feeling much more energetic by the end of it than I would have done sitting on the train and heading straight home. The exertion of any type of exercise actually tends to give you more energy rather than less – try it yourself, it's true!

So, from your list of exercise that you enjoy or would like to try, I want you to use the planner below to slot in when you will do this. I've lost count of the times people say they don't have time to exercise. This is simply not true and can be translated into, "exercising is not a priority for me" or "I don't really want to exercise".

By using the planner, you will be able to identify free times during your week when you can slot in a little exercise. I defy anyone to tell me that they don't have a free ten minutes where they can go out a short walk and build this up over time.

Depending on your current level of exercise, aim to increase it by ten minutes each day, or even five if ten seems like too much of a stretch. The recommended minimum level of exercise for an adult is thirty minutes of cardiovascular exercise at least five days a week, but if you are trying to lose weight, you will need to aim for a little more than this.

The more exercise you do, the more weight you will lose. But remember the key points – do something you enjoy, and fit it realistically around your schedule. If you have not exercised for a long time or have a health condition, then speak with your GP first. He or she may be able to suggest the best type of exercise to start with. In many areas there are exercise classes run specifically for people with various health conditions, such as heart disease or mobility problems, so speak to your GP about going along to these if you are worried about the impact of exercise on your health.

If you are really struggling to stick to your exercise plan, I'd suggest meeting up with other people, as this makes you more likely to stick to it and not make up excuses at the last minute. Why not go for a walk with a colleague at lunchtime, or join a local running group or exercise class with a friend?

Whilst I have my set ways for doing things which I find helpful, I have learned so many tips from speaking with other people, because everyone finds different techniques that work for them. Several people voiced how bored they get when walking any distance alone, so someone suggested downloading an audio book onto their MP3 player to listen to as they walked. This is an interesting alternative to music, although I find a playlist of upbeat music very motivating, too.

On days when you really can't be bothered exercising, read over your goal card again to visualise why you are putting yourself through it. Tell yourself that you are only going to exercise for five minutes, which should at least get you out and get you started. If you do only manage five minutes, then that is five minutes more than nothing. But I usually find that once I have started I can stretch that a little.

Keep telling yourself "just another five minutes" or "just to the end of that road, then the next road". It's amazing how easy it is to fool your own brain.

As an added incentive, when I'm exercising I like to imagine that the fat is melting off me as I walk, or if I'm at an exercise class I like to imagine the muscles toning up and becoming harder as I'm doing it. Really visualising the outcomes is the best incentive you can use to push yourself that little bit further. David Hamilton's book, How Your Mind Can Heal Your Body, has fantastic visualisations for many ailments, but I particularly like the ones related to losing weight. Take a look at it for inspiration.

Below is an example of an activity planner that you could use to make your exercise plan. First, cross out every box when you are in work or have other essential commitments, then you will be able to see at a glance how many boxes you actually have free. Plan your exercise in these free boxes at times that are easiest for you to stick to. On the next page I have completed one as an example:

	Monday	Tuesday	Wednesday	Thursday	Friday	Saturday	Sunday
6-7am	X	X	X	X	X	X	X
7-8am	X	X	X	X	X	X	X
8-9am	X	X	X	X	X	X	X
9-10am	X	X	X	X	X		
10-11am	X	X	X	X	X		House work
11-12 noon	X	X	X	X	X		House work
12-1pm	X	X	X	X	X	Shopping	
1-2pm	X	X	X	X	X	Shopping	
2-3pm	X	X	X	X	X	Cook	
3-4pm	X	X	X	X	X	Cook	
4-5pm	X	X	X	X	X		
5-6pm	Walk	Walk	Walk	Walk	Walk		
6-7pm							
7-8pm	Visit mum			cinema	Meet friends		
8-9pm	Visit mum			cinema	Meet friends		
9-10pm					Meet friends		
10-11pm					Meet friends		
11-midnight							

When I look at this plan, I see that I am free on a Tuesday and Wednesday evening and a Sunday afternoon. I also have time later on each evening when I could take five minutes to write out my meal plan or read my goal cards.

I know that I enjoy having time to myself on a Sunday, so I would not plan in any exercise for that day, and Saturdays are often busy so I couldn't commit regularly to a class then either, but I could check out what Zumba classes are available on Tuesday or Wednesday evenings and add that into my schedule.

This plan works for me, but other people might prefer to keep their weeknights free and go to an exercise class in their free time on the Saturday morning, for example. Play to your strengths and make the plan work for you. For example, if you have children, plan in going to the park and running around with them for an hour, or going swimming or cycling at the weekend. If you are busy every evening, then go for a walk or a run during your lunch break.

Fill out an activity planner for yourself now:

Your turn

	Monday	Tuesday	Wednesday	Thursday	Friday	Saturday	Sunday
6-7am							
7-8am							
8-9am							
9-10am							
10-11am							
11-12 noon							
12-1pm							
1-2pm							
2-3pm							
3-4pm							
4-5pm							
5-6pm							
6-7pm							
7-8pm							
8-9pm							
9-10pm							
10-11pm							
11-midnight							

Rather than viewing exercise as a chore, I'd like you to see it as a way of fast-tracking your goals and making yourself feel better, not worse.

Many people are used to doing as little exercise as possible. They park their car in the closest space to the door of the supermarket, or head straight for the lift rather than taking the stairs. All these little actions do add up and make a difference, because they are changing your mind-set as well as your body shape.

As well as the exercise you have scheduled in throughout your week, I would like you to look for every opportunity in your day to embrace physical activity rather than avoid it. This means automatically using the stairs rather than the lift, walking to the next bus stop or train station rather than plumping for the nearest one, or leaving the car at home when going somewhere local.

Could you march on the spot while waiting for the kettle to boil, or do some squats while running the bath? You will be amazed at how much more energetic you feel when using more energy.

> **Checklist**
>
> 1. Only do exercise you enjoy, that way you will stick to it.
>
> 2. Start with whatever you can manage and build it up.
>
> 3. Exercise has countless benefits, not just for your weight but in generally boosting your mood so it's worth a try.
>
> 4. Exercising with a friend can make you more likely to stick to the plan.
>
> 5. If you are really struggling to get out, read through your goal cards and imagine that excess fat slipping away.
>
> 6. Plan in exercise around your weekly commitments, but add in spontaneous exercise, too, whenever the opportunity arises.

Chapter 6

Coping with Cravings

It's everyone's downfall. You think: Right, I can do this plan, it's not so hard. You've been doing well all day and then BOOM! Out of nowhere a craving fills your head and it's all you can think about. That milky, smooth chocolate bar, the greasy, fatty bag of chips. Your brain tells you that you must have it, you can't cope without it, how will you carry on with the rest of your day if you don't get the object of your desire right now? Well, you can carry on just fine, actually. Don't panic, it's only a craving. Have you ever tried denying yourself the craving to see what actually happens? It's not as bad as you might imagine.

Notice that earlier I said that the craving fills your head. That's exactly where it fills. It is nothing to do with your stomach needing the food.

I'd like to explain the difference between different states of hunger. These are hunger, desire and cravings.

Hunger is an empty stomach. You feel physically hungry and it is time to eat. It's okay to eat when you are hungry; in fact, this is your body telling you that you should be eating now. It's the other two states that cause the problems and get us confused.

Desire is when you are not particularly hungry but you eat because there is food around. Maybe you are at a party and they put the buffet out, or someone has brought in a cake or biscuits to work. Had this food not been put in front of you, you would not have thought about eating at that time because you are not hungry. But now you've seen it, it's all you can think about and you want it.

A craving, on the other hand, is a thought that comes over you for no apparent reason. It fills your head and your taste buds with the thought of a particular type of food. So it's not just general hunger, because it is only one type of food that will do at that moment. I don't know about you, but I used to try and eat something else in response to the craving – something healthier, thinking that would be enough to get rid of it. But in the end I'd have eaten five healthier items and then still go back and get the object of my craving, too!

So to deal with these three states, it's first of all important to be able to identify them so that you know what you are dealing with. It is good practice before you eat anything to ask yourself: "How hungry am I right now?" Measure this on a scale of zero to ten, with ten being completely stuffed full (imagine that feeling after Christmas dinner); five is comfortable, neither particularly hungry or not hungry; and zero is starving, stomach completely empty.

You should only eat if your score is four or less. I know that scales like this are very subjective and it can be difficult to gain any real meaning from the numbers, but the object of the exercise is just getting you to tune into your hunger and only eat when you are actually hungry.

It sounds simple, but I can't tell you the amount of times I have eaten for many other reasons rather than actually being hungry, and I imagine you might be the same.

I used the example of the feeling of fullness after Christmas dinner. This is actually way over the limit of feeling full. You should never feel stuffed and uncomfortable after eating a meal. It means you have gone too far and should be avoided at all costs.

By eating mindfully, you should be more alert to when you are becoming full as you are giving the food time to register. Ask yourself: "Could I go for a brisk walk right now without feeling uncomfortable?" If you are unsure if you are getting full, stop and remind yourself that there is always another meal coming. We are lucky enough to live in a country where food is not in short supply, so there is no need to stuff in everything in sight now as if it is your last supper.

When you begin to feel full, stop and remind yourself that you can always go back and finish the rest if you are still hungry in twenty minutes so leave the remainder for now. If you are still hungry in twenty minutes, go back and eat a little more, but most likely you will find that you are no longer hungry.

Remember, food is fuel; it is necessary and even better if it is delicious, but it should only be taken when needed. You wouldn't continue to fill your car with petrol when it had reached its limit, would you?

So, what do you do when you know it's a craving or desire but you still really want it anyway? I'd like you to write a flashcard that you will keep in your pocket, purse, mobile phone, or wherever you can have instant access to it. This flashcard is a little affirmation or note to yourself to remind you that a craving is not a state of emergency and you can handle it.

The aim of this is to slow down your thinking so that you are not reacting irrationally to the thoughts. Something like "this is only a craving, it is not an emergency so I don't have to react" should do the job, but word it in a way that makes sense to you. This alone will not always be enough, but it gives you time to put the other techniques into action. So, next up:

Distraction, Distraction, Distraction. Put off eating for fifteen minutes, or even five minutes if that is all you can manage. Tell yourself that you can still have it if you want it after that time has passed. During that time, do another task to take your mind off the food.

If you are at work, tell yourself you will eat after you have made the next phone call or written another email. If you are at home, phone a friend, do a crossword, read a chapter of a book, or ideally paint your nails so that you physically can't go and get the food.

After you have completed whatever task you've set yourself, push yourself to wait another five minutes and do something else – make another call, check your emails, whatever. It's even better if you can do something that engages your mind so that you are not still thinking about the food during that time. For example, a Sudoku puzzle or crossword will focus your mind with no room for thoughts of food.

If you are in a situation where none of these distraction tasks are possible, then use your own mind and surroundings to distract you, as that is always available.

A friend of mine, Kevin Feeney, told me about the "I wonder" technique, which I just find fantastic in so many situations to distract myself from food, anxiety, worry, or any other type of troublesome thoughts. Practise it now. Wherever you are, look around you and ask the question: "I wonder..." about whatever catches your attention first. "I wonder where they bought that lampshade", "I wonder what the temperature is outside", "I wonder where he was born", "I wonder where she bought her jumper", "I wonder when this building was built". There are endless possibilities to wonder about. You don't need to find out the answer; in fact, you shouldn't find it out. It is enough just to wonder curiously, as this engages your brain and you will be surprised how quickly you forget what you were initially thinking or worrying about.

Another method is to take the mindfulness technique a bit further than just eating mindfully. Take a few deep breaths, by which I mean moving your breath down to your diaphragm, at the bottom of your rib cage, rather than just breathing shallowly in the top of your chest. You can check you are doing this by ideally lying down – sitting is okay, too – and putting one hand on your stomach and one hand on the top of your chest, in the middle, just under your collarbone. If you are breathing deeply, the hand on your stomach should be the only one moving in and out. You want it to move in and out as far as possible, whilst your hand on your chest should remain relatively still.

After taking a few of these deep breaths, start to notice your surroundings. Can you feel the seat underneath you or the ground beneath your feet? Is the chair hard or soft, warm or cold? Where does the chair touch your body? Can you feel it taking your weight underneath you, or can you feel it supporting your back? Maybe you are wearing a big woollen scarf or a light, floaty summer skirt. Can you feel the clothes against your skin?

Then move on to what you hear. Can you hear traffic outside or a clock ticking? Are there voices in the next room, or music playing nearby? Listen to each sound in turn, focussing your attention on that. Maybe you are somewhere with quite distinctive smells. If you are in a coffee shop, maybe you can smell the coffee aroma; if you are in a department store, can you smell the different perfumes and make up all around you? If you are in a park, can you smell the freshly cut grass, or if you are on the beach, can you smell suntan lotion?

Now what can you see in front of you? Is there a picture on the wall? Or a tree outside the window? Look at the branches, the leaves, the different colours and patterns. Are you outside? Focus on the clouds. The sky can be made up of fascinating colours and shapes of clouds that are always there but which we rarely notice as we rush about our busy lives. Take a moment to really look at them. As you do this, keep breathing deeply as you take in every detail around you.

Even as you read through that paragraph, I bet you have forgotten all about food. So try doing this whenever you get a craving. Not only will it make you forget all about your craving, but it is a very powerful technique to calm you and bring you back in control so that things don't seem quite as unachievable as before.

Lots of people find this type of mindfulness exercise or breathing relaxation very helpful to calm the mind, but other people prefer a muscle-based relaxation. This starts in the same way, by taking a few slow, deep breaths, then slowly turn your attention to each muscle group in turn.

Start at your feet. Curl up your toes as tightly as you can. Hold it for a few seconds then release. Now pull your feet up so that your toes are pointing towards the ceiling; you will feel the tension in your calf muscles. Hold for a few seconds, then release. Move up your leg to your thighs, clench the muscles tightly then release. Now your stomach, pull your belly button in towards your spine, hold, then release. Clench your fists as tightly as you can, focus all your attention on that sensation in your hands, hold, and then release. Pull your shoulders up towards your ears, hold, then release. Now clench your jaw as tightly as you can. Really feel the tension, then release. Moving up your face, furrow your eyebrows, hold as before then release.

If there are any parts of your body that still feel tense, go back and tense the muscles in that area again, hold for a few seconds and release. Finish by returning your attention to your breath, taking those slow deep breaths before returning your focus to your surroundings.

This is a full body relaxation which can take some time to complete. If you don't have time to do this regularly, even just picking the two or three areas where you know you hold the most tension can be helpful, and do a quick muscle relaxation focussing on these areas only. This can be less daunting to start with than a full body relaxation. It is often enough to calm your body and then your mind will naturally follow, as you cannot be both anxious and relaxed at the same time.

As you can imagine, these techniques are helpful in all sorts of situations, from public speaking to excessive worry, but in terms of weight loss they have just acted as a perfect distraction to thinking about food as well as putting you in a calmer frame of mind to deal with life's challenges, rather than reaching to food for comfort.

I know that I used to get very caught up in the fact that I didn't know how to breathe properly, or I didn't have time to do a full relaxation exercise. The thought of lying still and silent for an hour at a time filled me with horror and, quite frankly, it still does. But make mindfulness and relaxation work for you.

Some people will relish the idea of getting into a deep relaxational state but if, like myself, you are not one of them, then don't get hung up on it. Do what you can and what you feel comfortable with. If you are worrying too much about how you are breathing, then you are missing the point of relaxing. I am giving you pointers to aim for, but I purposefully never suggest that people count their breaths as this is something that people get hung up on if they can't breathe in or out for that set number of counts.

So, maybe in the beginning your stomach won't push out much when you breathe, but go with it for now and over time you may notice it expands that little bit more on your in-breaths. Similarly, people often give up relaxation like this when they can't seem to focus on the task at hand, because the thoughts they are trying to get away from keep slipping back into their mind. This is completely natural. Again, go with it. It's okay if that annoying thought sneaks back in. Acknowledge it – "there it is again" – and if you can, try and imagine it is inside a balloon and it naturally floats away out of your picture, or maybe imagine it as a cloud floating on by through the air. It was there, but now it's gone again. It might keep coming back for a while, but that's okay, it will float back out again.

Keep practising the mindfulness exercise above and it will become more manageable over time. Think of it like learning a language or learning to drive. I'm sure you weren't fantastic at either in the beginning, but with practice you may have mastered the skill a bit better.

Now I might be going against the teachings of many experts in the field of meditation and mindfulness here, but I'm writing this book to share my personal experience of losing weight with you.

So when it comes to practising relaxation, I do it in very short bursts as I truly believe that even a little does the world of good, compared to nothing at all. I don't want people to be put off by the thought of having to dedicate hours to it and then feeling disheartened when you can't fit it in or don't enjoy it.

I admit I really don't enjoy lying for even half an hour doing a relaxation, but I LOVE my short bursts of mindfulness which I find calm my mind hugely. So do whatever works for you. There are countless courses and books out there if you want to take up the practice of mindfulness or meditation, and if it interests you then I wholeheartedly suggest you go for it. It is so beneficial and you will have tutors who are much more practised in the art than myself. But for the purposes of losing weight and within this plan, I suggest practising the various relaxation exercises (above) when it suits you, and see what works best for you. That might be deep breathing while boiling the kettle, or some muscle relaxation while sitting on the bus.

You might find it strange that relaxation is included in a weight loss plan, but I see many reasons for doing so:

• It acts as a distraction technique to counteract cravings.

• It is a good technique for dealing with unwanted, negative emotions for those who comfort eat due to stress and anxiety.

• It brings people back into the "here and now" as this is all we can deal with, rather than worrying about what we ate yesterday or the enormity of our goals that we think we will never achieve.

• Relaxation boosts self-compassion, as it gives you time to slow things down and is a soothing activity.

After all, this approach is a whole, healthier lifestyle not just a quick fix to lose weight.

A final technique to deal with cravings is imagining how you will feel shortly after giving into them. Overeating, like any addiction, focusses on the short term gratification over long term gains. People who are successful in losing weight can swap this around and are ruled by the longer term gains over the short term good feelings.

Just before you go to eat that cake/chocolate bar/fish supper, imagine how you will feel ten minutes from now. Will you feel proud of yourself for having resisted temptation, or annoyed or disgusted with yourself for giving in? Visualise the restraint side of yourself versus the giving-in side of yourself. What does each side look like, sound like?

You need to practise building up your restraint muscle, as this will be your ally in fighting those cravings. Be familiar with it, so that it becomes a comfort as well as a motivator to your fight against over-eating. You also need to be aware of the giving-in muscle, so that you can recognise it as soon as it starts to encourage you to give in to the craving or not stick to your goals.

To do this, close your eyes and imagine that you have both a giving-in muscle and you have a restraint muscle. I use Judy Beck's image of a muscle here because I like to imagine building up a muscle and making it bigger, or alternatively not using it and it wastes away. But some people visualise it as a little conscience on either shoulder, like an angel and a devil.

Make up something that you can identify with, and starting with the giving-in muscle, I want you to imagine it. What does it look like? What colour is it? What does it smell like? What does it sound like when it speaks to you? Is it demanding, weak, sneaky, or is it a comfort to you? What does it say to you? Really connect with this image of your giving-in muscle. It has a big part to play in your relationship with food.

Now, let's move your giving-in muscle into the background of your mind for a little while. Bring your restraint muscle into the spotlight now and spend some time getting to know it. Again, what does it look like? What colour is it? What does it smell like? What does this muscle sound like when it speaks to you? Is it supportive, strong, and kind, or is it a little bossy or unknown to you? What does it say to you? Really connect with this image of your restraint muscle. It's important to start building a good relationship with it as you tackle your relationship with food, because it's on your side in this battle.

All of the techniques described in this chapter aim to give you a little bit of breathing (and thinking) space to stop you reacting in the heat of the moment and making a poor choice. Slowing down your thoughts allows you to make a more considered decision of whether to eat or not.

It's important to be realistic and realise that sometimes you will still go on to over-eat, even after distracting yourself, but these tools will work some of the time and the more you use them the more they will work.

If you can resist a craving even just 50% of the time, then that is still a lot of unnecessary calories saved.

Checklist

1. Label each hunger state as what it is: Actual hunger, desire, or craving.

2. Read your emergency craving flashcard: "It's not an emergency, it's only a craving that will pass shortly."

3. Use the distraction techniques listed to put off eating for fifteen minutes, or even five if that's all you can manage.

4. Use relaxation exercises to gain control when you are in the midst of a craving.

5. Short term versus long term gratification – imagine how you will feel after giving in to your craving.

Chapter 7

It's the Thought that Counts

Humans are such irrational creatures. Even those of us that appear rational and level-headed on the outside, tend to have a stream of irrational, crazy thoughts going on underneath the calm exterior. We assume our thoughts are true, but they are all made up in our head. Yes, they are based on our experience of the world, but that is exactly what makes them biased. That and the fact that we tend to be more focussed on the negative aspects of life. When we were still cavemen and women, it bene-fited us to focus on every threat that might come our way in order to survive for longer. But this "threat system" has not been dialled down enough for our modern lives, and so we are left still focus-sing on all the negatives and threats around us without taking equal consideration of the positives.

Always thinking negatively is not any more realistic than always thinking positively. Both have a chance of happening, so let's practise bringing our thoughts into some middle ground.

What's this got to do with losing weight, I hear you ask? Well, behaviour is not automatic; there is always a thought behind it. If we can take control of our thoughts, we can take control of the behaviour that follows. The main difference between successful, long term weight loss is the ability to think rationally and not go off track when you eat a few calories more than you'd planned to.

If we let our thoughts spiral out of control, we can easily go off track. Thoughts such as "what's the point?", "I've ruined it now", or "I'll start again on Monday", lead to over-eating. How often have you gone off track by eating something extra and then thought, "Well, I may as well keep eating now, I'll just order a takeaway for dinner and I'll start again on Monday."?

I would by no means describe myself as a completely rational thinker, even now. I think for everyone it is a work in progress, but I'm happy to say that I believe I am now a pretty rational thinker when it comes to eating (one day I'll get there with the rest of my life!).

As I write this book, I am enjoying a delicious lemon tart in my favourite coffee shop. I will enjoy it, I will finish it, and that is it over. I will not go home and order a takeaway and then tomorrow think I'll just keep eating everything in sight and start back on my diet when I go back to work on Monday.

I know many people that think this way and end up overeating for days (or weeks in a row), but that is why they put on weight. It is not the one cake they eat in the beginning that causes the weight gain.

I also have friends who think completely rationally about food and I have never heard them utter the words, "I shouldn't have eaten that burger", or "I can't believe I had a second helping of that trifle, I'm such a slob." It's not that they don't eat the burger or the trifle, they do. But they keep it in context, and you won't find them obsessing about what they have or have not eaten. Eating it now and again is not a problem.

Unsurprisingly, the friends I know who think in this way are all slim. Some people may say that is why they don't obsess about food, because they are already slim anyway. But what if I turn this on its head and say maybe they are slim because of their rational thinking when it comes to food? If we all thought rationally about food, would our behaviour not follow?

As a rule of thumb, it takes approximately 3,500 calories to put on 1lb in weight (Beck), so you have far from failed if you eat one slice of cake now and again. It's the sabotaging thoughts that follow that one slice of cake that lead to the weight gain. Until you get your irrational thoughts under control, it is worthwhile using a flashcard to help you get back on track. For example, my flashcard might say:

"It takes over 3,000 calories to put on 1lb in weight, so that extra I ate just now won't make a difference to my weight as long as I continue sticking to my plan from now on. No need to continue overeating, just get back on it now!"

This ability to get back on track quickly is the key difference between the common media notion of "thinking like a thin person" (Judy Beck), or being locked in a cycle of over-eating.

So firstly we need to identify what irrational thoughts sound like, before we can move onto challenging them and finally changing them. An irrational thought has several characteristics. It is:

• Negative towards yourself or others: "I'm so stupid."

• It is inflexible and rigid: "I must never eat cake again."

• It gets in the way of achieving your goals: "I've failed, I'll never lose weight."

• It is not based in reality: "If I starve myself all day, then I'll reach my target weight quicker."

Basically, it's unhelpful to you!

It helped me immensely to know that we all have negative thoughts. These are sometimes known as thinking errors, and fall into various categories. If you can identify your negative thought as one of these thinking errors, it is another piece of evidence to support the fact it is not necessarily true. And by labelling it as such, it can sometimes take the weight from it.

Thinking Errors

1. Catastrophising

Negative prediction – "I can't believe I ate that fish supper. I'm going to put on all the weight I just lost."

2. Labelling

Fixed generalised labels on self and others – "I'm so fat."

3. Mind reading

You assume that people are reacting negatively to you when you have no definite evidence for this – "Mary thinks I'm so rude for not eating the cake she baked."

4. Personalisation

You blame yourself for something you are not responsible for, i.e. other people's feelings – "If I don't eat dinner with my family then I will make them feel bad."

5. Shoulds and Musts

You criticise yourself and others using demanding rules – "I must never eat any sweets."

6. Discounting the positives

You dwell on the negatives, giving them more importance than the positives – "I've failed at the diet plan this week, I just couldn't stick to eating sitting down." (Discounting the fact that you did lots of exercise and practised relaxation.)

Over the next week, start identifying each time you have a thought like the ones above, and say to yourself, "There's me mind reading again", or "That's me catastrophising". Notice how it takes the power out of the thought, when you don't automatically assume it is true.

Imagine the scenario. You have been out for a lovely pub lunch, maybe you went for the homemade burger and chips and a lovely cheesecake for dessert. If you thought rationally you might come to the conclusion, "I can't eat healthily all the time", "It's no big deal", and you'd spend very little time actually thinking about the lunch after it was over; you would simply get on with the rest of your day.

However, if you think irrationally about food, you might be very hard on yourself, call yourself names, etc, and the likelihood is you would spend a lot longer thinking about the lunch you've just eaten because you are over-estimating the damage that it has done so it will have a knock-on effect for how you eat for the rest of the day, or even week.

Most of us have been programmed to think that you must be harsh on yourself if you want to lose weight, but that will simply lock you into an unhelpful cycle of being annoyed with yourself, over-estimating the damage you have done, and therefore eating more either for comfort or to rebel against the strict boundaries you have placed on yourself.

In order to catch these negative thoughts, ask yourself, "What was just going through my mind?" Ask this either the second you start to notice you are feeling bad, or right before you pick up another piece of food. List these thoughts. As you look back over this list, keep in mind the key question: "Is this thought helpful to me?"

If it's not, then it has no use floating around your head and it's time to get rid of it. I'm sure you've heard this before, but would you say these things to a friend? What is the actual evidence to support this thought? What evidence do you have against this thought? Imagine yourself as a High Court judge, and go through the following example:

Real Life Example

"I've just eaten that huge big lunch at the pub. I'll never lose weight now."

The first sentence is true, therefore you can't challenge it, so let's focus on the second sentence, which is the part that is actually upsetting us and leading into this cycle of overeating.

What is the evidence that you will never lose weight?

1. I didn't stick to my plan today.

What is the evidence that this thought may not be true?

1. I've lost weight before.

2. I have all these new CBT techniques to try that I haven't known about before.

3. I know for a fact that the meal maybe consisted of 1000 calories, which in itself is not enough to lead to ongoing weight gain forever.

4. It is an example of catastrophizing.

Now look at your evidence for and against your negative thought. Using both sides of the argument, is there something that you could say to yourself that is more helpful and realistic instead of "I'll never lose weight"? Because, remember, "I'll never lose weight" is not a fact, it is just a thought you have made up in your head. So let's make up another one instead. It might go something along the lines of:

"Although I ate more than I'd planned to today, I have all the skills and techniques available to me to lose weight, and one blip cannot foretell the outcome of my weight loss plan"

Your Turn:

Negative thought:

Evidence that confirms this thought:

Evidence against this thought (including what type of thinking error it is):

```



```

Alternative, more realistic thought:

```



```

Learning to identify and challenge your faulty thinking is a skill, and like all skills it takes time and practice to learn. If these techniques sound cumbersome, remember you will eventually do them automatically without thinking. If you can drive, remember that first driving lesson when everything was new and it took a lot of concentration. Now you probably don't even remember how you got from A to B most of the time, because you drive without even thinking about the skills involved; it's become part of your unconscious now. The same eventually happens with any new skill we learn.

The thought patterns we have been talking about in this chapter are usually quite easy for us to access in our heads. We all have many of them floating in and out constantly through the day; some we are aware of, and some we are not. In the next chapter we are going to delve a little further to reach our underlying beliefs, which shape our behaviour and choices even more.

Checklist

1. Start identifying the thought that occurs right before eating, or the nasty things you say to yourself after over-eating.

2. Label each thought as the appropriate thinking error.

3. Start challenging your negative thoughts by questioning the evidence for and against its truth.

4. Start saying the new, more realistic thought to yourself in place of the old negative thought. You made up the original negative thought in your head, so what's the difference in making up a more realistic one?

5. Getting back on track instantly after a slip-up is the key to successful weight loss.

6. Remember thoughts are not facts!

Chapter 8

Updating Your Instruction Manual

If you can imagine our core beliefs are a bit like our instruction manual or guidebook, they inform everything we do so to change our eating habits, we must form new beliefs around weight loss and food in order to sustain long term change. This is where we really fundamentally start to differ from other weight loss plans because changing our core beliefs and rules about food is like changing our instruction manual on how we live our life. Therefore new eating habits start to become ingrained and part of a new lifestyle. It is no longer viewed as short term diet but a better way of living.

Our underlying beliefs have usually been around since childhood but are sometimes shaped by a big, life-changing event later on in life too. I realised our beliefs had an impact on eating habits when I would ask people to go home and resist eating part of the food on their plate. They found this exercise of throwing away a small amount of food from their plate one of the most difficult parts of the programme. The reason for this is because we all have these beliefs guiding our behaviour (sometimes we are not even aware of them) and quite often when it comes to food it is lessons we have learned from our parents when we were small regarding wasting food and needing to finish everything on your plate which makes it almost impossible for some people to only eat what they want and leave the rest.

I ask people to practice this resistance exercise for times when they are eating out and have no control over the portion sizes. Try it tonight – overfill your plate with food and only eat the amount that you section off according to your usual portion size. I am only asking you to do this one time, it will not be a regular exercise as obviously wasting food for the sake of it is something to be avoided.

To help you resist the remaining food:

- Ask yourself "how will I feel in ten minutes if I resist this food or if I eat it?"

- Recite in your head the reasons you are doing this i.e. your reasons for losing weight

If you found it difficult to throw the food away, you need to be aware of what beliefs were getting in the way. Ask yourself the following:

- What rules did you learn in childhood regarding food?

- Whose rules are they?

- How useful are they to you now?

For example, I was told when I was a child:

"What a waste! Why do I bother going to all that trouble?"

"There are starving children in Africa who would love to eat this!"

"If you don't finish your dinner you won't get any dessert"

I am not trying to make you blame your parents here. Parents do the best they can and say these things to try to encourage their picky children to eat more to gain the nutrition that they need to grow. This is necessary when you are a child but you don't need to live by these same rules when you are an adult. You are now in charge of what to put into your body and in fact holding on to the same rules from childhood can be counter-productive in adulthood. For example:

"What a waste! Why do I bother going to all that trouble?" is using the emotion of guilt to encourage people to eat. Listen to your body and eat if you are hungry, not for any other reason.

"There are starving children in Africa who would love to eat this!" – this is a fact, but it is irrelevant to how much you should eat. If you want to help starving children, donate food to a food bank or money to charity, don't force feed yourself as that won't solve the problem of other people starving in the world.

"If you don't finish your dinner you won't get any dessert" – whilst this may be helpful to give children a nutritionally balanced diet and ideally adults would follow a healthy, balanced diet too, if you are going to eat a pudding anyway, there is really no point in forcing down the main course just so you can force down a pudding too and feel over full. Why not reduce the portion sizes of both to allow you to eat it?

These responses to my rules are written from a rational, adult perspective which is much more helpful for losing weight than continuing to follow out of date rules from childhood unquestioningly. Now you have a go. Remember your new rules are yours alone, you can make up what you like to suit your lifestyle and goals.

Your Turn

Old Rules

·

·

·

New Rules

·

·

·

The previous rules were ones we learned in childhood, but you may also find that you live by another set of rules which you have placed upon yourself in line with what you think an overweight person should or should not do. Many people have been over-weight for so long that they cannot imagine being any other way. They live their life according to the box they have placed themselves in.

I have heard many people say that they couldn't possibly go to the gym or go on holiday, for example, because they would feel embarrassed working out next to slimmer people or wouldn't feel comfortable wearing "summer clothes" or a swimsuit at their current size. This is a very limiting mind-set and only comes about from your own made-up rules. Why place these restrictions on your life just because of your size?

When we continue to hold negative beliefs about ourselves or our situation, we become stuck and it's harder to move forward. Many people put their lives on hold until they reach their elusive perfect weight. What are you putting on hold?

1.

2.

3.

4.

5.

Why are you waiting? Why can you only do these things at a certain weight? What do you think will be so different about being thinner? What will you have that you don't believe you have now?

Read over your list and pick something you can do this week. If that seems too big a step, then break each item down into smaller goals. For instance, if you've been putting off joining a gym then why don't you research different gyms in your area first, then check out the prices, then maybe go for a trial session before committing to joining? By changing your behaviour, your mind-set will follow.

If you have nothing to add to this list then it's great that you are not putting your life on hold until you become slimmer. Sadly, though, a lot of people don't do things because they feel too big to do them or they feel they will be better at them or have more confidence after they have lost weight, i.e. join an exercise class, go out dancing more, wear nice clothes.

It really is true that if you fake it at first, you will eventually feel confident in acting that way so start today "acting as if" you have already lost the weight, and positive change will follow.

Now, let's imagine for a moment that you are not overweight any more. You are already your ideal weight. How would your life be different if you were slimmer? Take a few moments to answer the following questions. Go with your instinct, don't overthink the answers!

What would you be doing differently?

How would you spend your free time?

How would other people react towards you?

How would you feel towards yourself?

```
┌────────────────────────────────────────────────┐
│                                                  │
│                                                  │
│                                                  │
│                                                  │
└────────────────────────────────────────────────┘
```

This exercise may help you to really visualise why you want to lose weight, and if you can visualise it then you can do it. "You can't do what you can't imagine" because you don't even know it exists. If you have always been overweight or for a very long time, you may have lost sight of it even being possible for you to be any other way.

Wherever we place our attention is what becomes our biggest focus. So if you think and talk constantly about the problems you have, then this is what your life becomes. If you spent that same amount of time focussing on the solutions, rather than going over and over the problem, the solution would become the bigger part of your life. Always remember - wherever we place our attention is what we become. See David Hamilton's work for more scientific research on this concept.

By imagining what it is like to be slim, you have something to work towards and you will find yourself naturally veering towards acting like a slimmer person. We invest a lot of time and effort in trying to prove ourselves right. If we tell ourselves we are over-weight and will always be that way, then it is counter-intuitive to actually lose the weight and prove ourselves wrong. It's the same for any belief we hold. Think of someone who has a core belief of "I'm a failure". They will be more alert to all the evidence in their life that supports this belief, whilst generally ignoring the evidence against this view because it doesn't fit in with what they have been telling themselves. Even though it is uncomfortable to view ourselves as a failure or overweight or any other negative belief we hold about ourselves, we cling onto it because generally humans don't like change. So we don't know how to act when we start telling ourselves that the opposite is true.

As with everything, it takes practice and repetition to start believing it. In the beginning it can be a step too far to replace your negative beliefs with the complete opposite. So turning "I'm a failure" into "I'm fantastic and perfect at everything" is equally unrealistic. What about "I'm okay" or "I'm good enough". Or with your weight, instead of the horrible names many people call themselves such as "I'm a fat pig"; maybe you could try "I'm on my way to being slimmer".

Remember the 5 factor model we discussed earlier in the book. By making a change to any one factor, the others will follow. Doing things now, instead of putting them off until you are a certain weight, will prove to yourself that you can be that person you want to be. It might feel strange at first, but fake it until you make it!

Checklist

1. Think about the rules you heard when you were a child regarding finishing your dinner.

2. Practise resisting food so that you learn that you don't need to finish everything on your plate.

3. Challenge your childhood rules by replacing them with more realistic ones from an adult's point of view.

4. Being able to visualise how your life will be when you are slimmer focuses your mind on getting there.

5. Don't put things off until you have lost weight. Live life now and your ideal weight will follow.

Chapter 9

Emotional Eating

Stress, boredom, anxiety, anger, sadness. I eat in response to all of these emotions. Like any addiction, overeating tends to take over when we are experiencing any type of negative emotion. As my counselling studies tutor once told us, "The suppression of expression leads to depression." Think of it like an emotion is building up inside of you. Maybe this is a sense of sadness or hopelessness, fear or worry. Instead of sitting with this emotion and really feeling it, the easier option is to push it down deep inside of you and hope that it will disappear.

For emotional eaters, the food acts as the suppressant but other common suppressants you might be familiar with are alcohol, cigarettes, shopping, gambling or taking drugs (I use the term "suppressant" here to mean a substance which pushes your emotions down, not a particular drug with a suppressing effect, as some drugs are obviously stimulants rather than suppressants).

With each of these unhelpful behaviours you are aiming to push down your feelings to avoid dealing with them. Unfortunately, however, by pushing them down you are only making them more ingrained inside you. They have to be let out rather than kept in, in order for them to be dealt with and then released. If you know that you are avoiding some deep-rooted problem that has been plaguing you for some time, I suggest you speak with a therapist if you can, as some people really benefit from this type of support to work through their issues.

Some people go off food during difficult times, and you may be someone who eats more in good times. Either way, it's essential to remember that food is fuel. It is not a helpful response to any other situation apart from physical hunger. The trick is to think up more useful responses to each emotion before they occur so that you are ready for them, rather than relying on food to get you through each one.

Emotions are banded about all the time, but have you ever taken a moment to think what each one actually feels like for you? Where do you feel it in your body? What thoughts are present? How does it make you behave/act? For example, if I am anxious, I can feel my stomach clenching and knotting, I might become light-headed and unable to concentrate. My thoughts start to spiral out of control, thoughts like "What if?", "I'll never cope with this…", "It will be unbearable", fly through my head.

In the past, I would have eaten something because I love food and it brought me some comfort. However, this comfort would be short-lived as it wasn't dealing with the source of the anxiety. If I actually challenged these negative thoughts (like I described in previous chapters) or if I did a short relaxation in the form of focussing on my breathing and slowing my body down, I would begin to feel calmer without the need for food. This in turn would take away the second round of negative emotions later when I became upset at myself for over-eating.

Take a few minutes now to really think what each emotion feels like to you. Think back to a time recently when you felt worried, sad, angry, anxious, scared or lonely. Can you remember physically how you felt? Was your stomach churning, were your shoulders tense, was your head spinning, did you feel sick, or did you feel empty, deflated or have a heavy heart or sinking feeling in your stomach?

Everybody is different, so there are no right or wrong answers here. But it is important to know what each emotion feels like and be able to name it, so that when it occurs you can spot the first signs of it before it becomes overwhelming. Some people find this very difficult, but until you can recognise anxiety, loneliness, sadness or fear inside yourself, how can you deal with it correctly?

If you are struggling with this exercise right now, then just be aware over the next few weeks any time you have a negative or even niggling feeling. Don't eat in response to it, but instead stop and really feel it so that you can identify what it is.

Now that you have identified various negative emotions within yourself, I would like you to come up with a plan to deal with them which does not include over-eating or any other addictive behaviours that you'd usually use to suppress them.

Complete the following plan of action so that you are better prepared with correct responses to each of the emotions listed below:

Next time I am scared I will ...

Next time I am anxious I will ...

Next time I am angry I will ...

Next time I am worried I will ...

```



```

Next time I am bored I will ...

```



```

Next time I am lonely I will ...

```



```

Next time I am sad I will ...

```



```

Next time I am stressed I will ...

```



```

Hopefully, by now you will realise that eating in response to each of these emotions will only make you feel better for a few minutes, but it does not deal with the actual problem. Furthermore, eating in response to any of these emotions actually leads to the secondary problem of feeling bad about yourself for over-eating!

Stop the vicious cycle now. When you are bored, do something enjoyable –read a book, plan something fun to do at the weekend. If you are anxious, focus on your breathing and calm your body down first, then challenge your negative thoughts. If you are lonely, phone a friend or send a wee text or email to someone you haven't heard from in a while.

My motto is "feel it and then deal with it". It's okay and natural to feel all of these emotions at times. Be aware of the feeling, acknowledge that it is okay, and then put a plan into action to deal with it and move forward. It is us who keep ourselves stuck in negativity. Our own thoughts keep fuelling anxiety and worry, our own behaviour keeps us bored or lonely. But that is great news, because it means that we are the ones who can change this and pull ourselves out of the repetitive, negative cycle.

I am not saying that it is easy to do but it can be done, and I have countless examples of people who have successfully dealt with emotions that were holding them back. Don't be disheartened when you have an off day; just get right back on track.

Self-esteem is another issue which can be intertwined with some people's weight gain. However, I'd like to note that this is not the case in every situation. Not everyone who is overweight suffers from low self-esteem, and certainly not everyone who is slim has high self-esteem. I raise the issue now, not only to offer a few pointers, but to make you aware that when we have low self-esteem change can seem impossible. We can only make lasting change when we feel good about ourselves, otherwise you will not feel you are worth making the time and effort for.

It is also important that if your self-esteem is low, you start to work on it now, not after you have lost weight. If you assume you will have sky high self-esteem once you have reached your ideal weight, you may be sorely disappointed.

For a more in-depth approach to improving self-esteem, I suggest you read the experts' opinion on this. Melanie Fennell's Overcoming Low Self-esteem is an excellent starting point.

There is not the scope here to go into the issue in-depth, but there are a few things you can do straight away to start raising your self-esteem. Firstly, I'd like to explain what I understand self-esteem to be, as it is such an over-used word that I think most people don't truly know the meaning of it. I think Dr David Burns has a lovely way of describing self-esteem as "the capacity to like and respect yourself when you lose, just as much as when you win".

Self-esteem is an opinion; it is not a fact, as our beliefs can be biased or inaccurate. And it is these negative beliefs about ourselves which underpin low self-esteem.

Beliefs develop as a consequence of your experiences in life. This can be early experiences as a child, or events in later life such as an abusive relationship, bullying in the workplace, or a traumatic event. So someone could have had a positive childhood and have quite high self-esteem, but a traumatic event later on could then have an impact on their current sense of themself. I wonder if you would judge someone else who'd had your experiences as negatively as you do yourself.

If we can get into the habit of rating our traits, not ourselves, this can help. Many people believe there is no such thing as a good or bad person, it's only their behaviours which are positive or negative. Not everyone agrees on this theory of human personality, of course, but even if you don't believe that there are no truly bad people in the world, I would imagine that most of you reading this book have not done anything truly awful in your life so there is no basis in rating yourself as a bad person.

Another common myth about self-esteem is that you either have high or low self-esteem and that's it. But it is not a fixed entity; it can and does go up and down, sometimes from week to week, sometimes from hour to hour! We can therefore make it go up more frequently by making subtle changes to our thought processes and behaviours. The reason I'm focussing on this here is that although self-esteem is dependent on many things, to be happy with yourself simply for existing puts you in a far stronger position to deal with life's challenges; challenges like losing weight.

How many times have you heard people say that they started a diet or gave up smoking/drinking but went off track as soon as something negative happened? To prevent all your good work being destroyed by an external event, it is useful to know your strengths, as these are part of you whatever situation arises. We are all too focussed on our weaker characteristics and what we are not good at, but looking at our positives boosts self-esteem as well as making us aware of all the skills we possess to cope in any given situation.

Look at the list below and, with a highlighter pen, I would like you to mark all the words that could apply to you. You do not have to be funny/hardworking/inquisitive 100% of the time – no-one inhabits their positive characteristics all of the time – but if you possess the characteristic even a little bit, then highlight it. Feel free to add any additional skills or characteristics to the list, as it is not exhaustive.

My Personal Strengths and Talents

Please highlight these from the list below

Dignified	Courageous	Curious
Inventive	Ambitious	Verbal
Prudent	Stable	Persevering
Intelligent	Imaginative	Trustworthy
Emotional	Loyal	Reflective
Energetic	Mature	Relaxed
Humorous	Patient	Spontaneous
Uninhibited	Fair-minded	Methodical
Reliable	Sensitive	Polite
Affectionate	Tough	Realistic
Trusting	Independent	Outgoing
Helpful	Sincere	Natural

Robust	Healthy	Funny
Obliging	Easy going	Open-minded
Friendly	Self-controlled	Generous
Opportunistic	Sensible	Optimistic
Organised	Hard working	Firm
Careful	Rational	Attractive
Responsible	Honest	Loving
Supportive	Assertive	Calm
Motivated	Confident	Bold
Strong	Warm	Considerate
Empathic	Flexible	Efficient
Practical	Tolerant	Likable
Capable	Charming	Cheerful
Competitive	Tactful	Witty
Creative	Thoughtful	Wise
Adventurous	Academic	Determined
Eager	Quiet	

Good at/with...

Managing money	Listening	Cooking
DIY	Exercise	Problem solving
Public speaking	Dancing	Trying new things
Art	Making decisions	Computers

(Exercise developed by Kevin Feeney)

Before doing this exercise, if I had asked you to name five positive qualities or characteristics you possess, I bet you would have found it extremely difficult. But I'm certain that you have marked more than five from the list above.

At first glance you might not have considered some of the words to be positive, for example "competitive", but this shows you that having a certain amount of competitiveness can be positive, it's just that we are so focussed on switching everything to negative that we don't realise it.

What has all this got to do with losing weight? Well, firstly, I wonder if you feel a little more positive about yourself knowing that you possess all those fantastic qualities. This is a starting point to lifting your self-esteem. Secondly, if you are aware of all the skills and qualities you possess, then whenever a tricky situation arises you can be more aware of your ability to cope without over-eating.

Some people have been overweight for so long that they cannot imagine being any other way. They have built their whole persona around being overweight and they attribute characteristics to the state of being "fat" or "thin".

I'd like you to make a note of all the words that come to mind when I say the word "fat" to you. List them under the word below. Don't think too much, just say the first word that comes to mind. Now do the same for the word thin.

Fat   Thin

It is so common for people to attribute characteristics to the word, which gives it much more power than it actually has. Common responses I have come across have included:

Fat = jolly, nurturing, warm or lazy, ugly, slob.

Thin = attractive, in control, happy or miserable, bony, cold.

If the words are negative down the fat side, no wonder your self-esteem takes a dip when you are overweight. On the other hand, if the words are positive on the fat side, maybe you find it hard to lose weight as you fear losing these good parts of yourself.

If your words are positive for thin and you are currently not as slim as you would like, it is denting your self-esteem to consider those who are thinner than you in these positive terms because you don't relate yourself to that. If your words are negative for thin, maybe you think you are going to develop all these negative characteristics if you lose weight.

Regardless of the way people couch the terms fat and thin, you are attributing actual characteristics to your weight, whether that weight is larger or smaller than you want to be. Weight does not have its own personality traits. For example, is every overweight person lazy? Or is every thin person mean? Are you really going to change your whole personality by losing or gaining a few pounds?

Both these words are extreme and negative, as it's not ideal to be either too fat or too thin, and I have purposefully used these words here to spark some emotional response. You need to think of a healthy weight in the middle of these two terms, where you can keep the personality traits you want to, and lose the negative ones that you associate with each state. I suggest the word "slim" or "healthy" to place in the middle of the line. What characteristics would that ideal weight have?

The next exercise is designed to explore how you truly feel about yourself, both when you are overweight and when you are thinner. You may find some interesting answers about how you view yourself as a person, simply by how much you weigh. Again, don't think too much about the answers, go with your gut instinct and the first answer that pops into your head.

Firstly, get into your overweight mind-set (most likely that's where you are right now anyway) and quickly complete the following statements:

When I'm overweight I _

When I'm socialising I _

When I'm by myself I _

When I'm overweight I can _

My clothes are _

When I'm overweight I stop _

When I'm overweight I start ‗

```
┌─────────────────────────────────────────┐
│                                           │
│                                           │
│                                           │
│                                           │
└─────────────────────────────────────────┘
```

Now let's imagine the slimmer version of yourself. Complete the following statements quickly, as if you were already at your ideal weight:

When I'm slim I ‗

```
┌─────────────────────────────────────────┐
│                                           │
│                                           │
│                                           │
│                                           │
└─────────────────────────────────────────┘
```

When I'm socialising I ‗

```
┌─────────────────────────────────────────┐
│                                           │
│                                           │
│                                           │
│                                           │
└─────────────────────────────────────────┘
```

When I'm by myself I ‗

```
┌─────────────────────────────────────────┐
│                                           │
│                                           │
│                                           │
│                                           │
└─────────────────────────────────────────┘
```

When I'm slim I can ‗

```
┌─────────────────────────────────────────┐
│                                           │
│                                           │
│                                           │
│                                           │
└─────────────────────────────────────────┘
```

My clothes are ‗

```
┌─────────────────────────────────────────┐
│                                           │
│                                           │
│                                           │
│                                           │
└─────────────────────────────────────────┘
```

When I'm slim I stop ..

```


```

When I'm slim I start ..

```


```

If you have found that you act and feel differently when you are overweight or slim, I'd like you to start acting and feeling like that slim person now. Right now! Don't put things off; don't feel inferior or awkward about your weight. Get into the mind-set of the slim you, and when you start acting in that way your weight will follow.

To help you practise acting like this confident, assured, slimmer version of yourself, you need to become more aware of all the undermining self-talk you are doing at present. Awareness is the first step to change, so from this moment on I want you to catch yourself every time you put yourself down, say you can't do something, or tell yourself that you are incapable of learning anything new, etc. On these occasions, ask yourself: "Is this helpful?"

On the other hand, if you tend to overeat in response to a happy situation, it is just as important to tune into why you are happy and enjoy the positive emotions in that moment rather than only focussing on eating. Whilst over-indulgence is part of many good times for people, a holiday or party or other celebration is about so much more than the food and drink. So focus on all the reasons you are so happy at that moment – quality time with friends, complete relaxation away from work, new places to visit, and things to experience. Start focussing on all these parts of the experience and immerse yourself in them.

Checklist

1. "Suppression of expression leads to depression" – start noticing your emotions and get them out in the open.

2. Tackle low self-esteem now, don't assume it will improve after you've lost weight.

3. Focus on your qualities and strengths, it's more helpful than focussing on your weaknesses.

4. Start acting like the slim version of yourself now and your weight will follow.

5. Our emotions exist to tell us that something is not right. Learn to listen to them and respond appropriately to deal with the issue.

Chapter 10

Dealing with Tricky Situations

I see many people losing weight using a lot of these techniques. Then a few months later some of them will tell me they have put weight on again. When I ask why, the common response is, "It was all going really well and then my boyfriend left me/work was really stressful/family are driving me mad."

This tells me instantly that they had been using some of the techniques but had missed out the section about really exploring their emotions. They think they don't need to delve into their emotions; after all, they only want to lose weight. But these excuses I have written above are classic examples of emotional eating.

Eating a box of doughnuts or a tub of ice-cream every day for a month will not bring your boyfriend back/give you a less stressful workplace/sort out your dysfunctional family, therefore eating is an unhelpful response to any of those situations. When we use unhelpful responses, they do nothing to sort the first problem and in addition they give us a secondary problem to deal with – putting on weight. Although that ice cream gives you a very short burst of comfort or even happiness, it is so short-lived is it really worth it?

If you see yourself in this scenario, go back through the chapter on dealing with emotions. It might also be helpful to read the chapter on thoughts, as sometimes people find it easier to tune into their thoughts and then the thoughts will lead you to your emotions if you are struggling to name them instantly. A handy tip to remember when trying to differentiate between your thoughts and emotions: An emotion is always one word only, whereas a thought tends to be more like a phrase:

Emotion – fear, anxiety, worry

Thought – "I will never lose weight."

On the other hand, people might cite Christmas, birthdays or holidays as their reason for piling on weight. I will say, first of all, that it is perfectly acceptable to put on a few pounds when on holiday or over Christmas. When I say a few pounds, I would allow myself to put on about 4lbs during these times and not worry about it.

The key point here is to remember that it is not a catastrophe to put on a little weight on holiday. Holidays are a time of enjoyment, of eating out more, maybe drinking a little more than usual. Standing on the scales after a holiday is the perfect situation in which to practise compassion on yourself, because it is this realistic compassion that will allow you to get instantly back on track. If you dissolve into a self-blaming, punitive mode, all you are doing is carrying on the over-eating because you feel bad, think it's a hopeless cause, and continue eating to make yourself feel better.

You've been on holiday and you've put on a couple of pounds, now get over it and get back on track as usual. There is no need to go on one of your old extreme diets to lose this excess weight. If you continue following the techniques as usual, the weight will come off slowly and steadily as before.

However, I have found since making these changes that I have seldom actually put on any weight whilst on holiday, because I continue with a lot of the techniques such as eating mindfully and only eating when sitting down. Of course I don't plan my meals when on holiday, but by keeping up as many of the techniques as possible, you will minimise any damage caused.

I can hear people complaining at this point and saying, "But I'm on holiday, I don't want to think about my weight" and whilst I agree that you shouldn't deprive yourself while on holiday, it is not a hardship to continue to eat mindfully. In fact, you have more time on holiday to enjoy your food, and it's lovely to really taste all these different cuisines and savour them as part of the distinctive holiday experience.

As is the case at home, when you eat mindfully you will naturally become aware of when you feel full and will stop eating much quicker because you have been more aware of what you have put into your body. Another positive aspect of being on holiday is that you can add in some exercise that you really enjoy, without it feeling like a chore. For example, is it really so horrible to take a walk along a sandy beach or lush, green park, or swim in the sea with the sun beating down on your skin, or dance the night away with friends? In fact, these are some of the things I relish most about going on holiday and it still counts as exercise.

So while you might say you don't have time when you are at home, you have all the time in the world when you are on holiday to indulge in these fun activities that are burning the excess calories you might be taking in.

Eating Out Tips

I have always maintained that I did not have to give up going out and enjoying myself when I lost weight. If I'd had to give up eating out, I wouldn't have succeeded. Everything in life is about balance and compromise, and that is the approach that is needed here, too. I still regularly go out for dinner and visit coffee shops with friends. These are really important aspects of my life but so, too, is being a healthy weight. Here are a few good tips which allow me to do both:

- Stick to two courses rather than three.

- Separate food on your plate to stay in keeping with portion size at home – you don't have to finish the whole plate.

- Continue to eat mindfully.

- Put your napkin on your plate to signal you are finished and can't go back to it, or even better, ask the waiter to take it away from the table if possible.

- Don't feel bad, start back on the plan immediately.

Why not ask for a half-sized portion for your main course if you know the portions are really big in your favourite restaurant? If you are out for someone's birthday, it is probably enough to have a small slice of birthday cake instead of dessert – not both! Remember, no food is off limits on this plan, but by eating a little bit less of everything you can still enjoy eating out and still have all your favourite foods.

While many people become more aware of what they are eating, often what they are drinking goes completely unchecked. It is important to be aware that drinks contribute to weight gain, too, whether that is alcohol or a syrup-loaded, milky, mega-sized coffee. Can you cut back on this a little without hindering your enjoyment? For example, could you order a smaller sized coffee, ask for skimmed milk instead of full fat, and hold back on syrup or whipped cream? Could you alternate your alcoholic drink with a glass of water, which will not only help your waistline but you'll wake up the next morning feeling much better? You will notice that everything I suggest here are just small adjustments – nothing drastic – but they all make a difference and, more importantly, ensure you will stick to the changes.

Forceful Feeders!

Some people struggle to say no to certain individuals. These individuals might be classed as "forceful feeders". You know the ones who always want you to have another biscuit or another helping of dinner, and don't seem to take no for an answer. My grandmother was definitely a forceful feeder; in fact, I think both my grandmothers were! Although I struggle with all the other issues covered in this book, luckily for me this is one area with which I never had a particular problem. I never felt guilty about declining food if I didn't want it, but I have come across many people who do find it difficult, so I thought it was worth discussing it here for those who struggle with "feeders".

A couple of important points:

You are not going to change these people; the change must come from you.

We often over-estimate the hurt we will cause by saying no to someone.

Disappointment is a normal part of life; it is not a tragedy for someone to feel disappointed if you don't eat their food, but frankly, I wouldn't feel in the least bit disappointed if someone didn't eat what I offered them, so their reaction says more about the person offering it than about you.

Think for a moment about how offended you would be if someone didn't eat all the food you gave them? Would you even remember tomorrow? I know I wouldn't even remember five minutes later.

You are not in charge of the other person's feelings, and in the grand scheme of things it is not such a big deal to refuse their offering.

Always ask yourself, "Is the other person's desire to have you eat more important than your desire to lose weight?"

Let's expand on this a bit more. If you were a vegetarian, would you eat meat just to please someone? I doubt it, so what is the difference between following a vegetarian diet and a diet of your own making to meet your own goals? It would suggest that you do not view your weight loss plan as legitimate as that of a vegetarian's diet, and therefore you do not view your life choices as important as other people's.

As a society we are often urged to put other people's needs first and quell our own desires. It can take some practice to be more assertive in order to state and stick by our needs in any situation, but it is important that you learn to do this if you are to succeed with your goals – in all areas of life, not just over-eating.

Read over the following list of statements and think about them in relation to your eating habits, particularly around other people.

1. You have the right to offer no reasons or excuses for justifying your behaviour.

2. You have the right to change your mind.

3. You have the right to make mistakes – and be responsible for them.

4. You have the right to say yes or no without feeling guilty or selfish.

5. You have the right to ask for what you want while accepting that asking doesn't always mean getting.

6. You have the right to be listened to and taken seriously.

7. You have the right to set your own priorities and state your own needs.

Extracted from Glasgow Gates "Bill of Rights"

If we don't apply these basic rights to ourselves, we can be left beating ourselves up when we don't meet them. And that leads into the vicious cycle of feeling bad about ourselves and eating for comfort, leading to lower self-esteem.

Below are examples of how these might convert into more assertive behaviours to assist in your weight loss.

1. You have the right to offer no reasons or excuses for justifying your behaviour.

If you want to stay off the alcohol on a night out to save on some calories, or just generally don't fancy any, then you don't need to justify this decision by saying, "I'm driving early in the morning", or "I'm taking antibiotics", or any other excuse that people use. Just say, "No thanks." People will soon forget it and move on.

2. You have the right to change your mind.

You can say initially that you will not eat any dessert when out, but may well change your mind by the end of the meal. This is okay.

3. You have the right to make mistakes – and be responsible for them.

Maybe you veered way off-plan one day and completely gave into your cravings. Everyone makes mistakes. Take responsibility, move on, and don't beat yourself up about it.

4. You have the right to say yes or no without feeling guilty or selfish.

So say "no thanks" to those forceful feeders who are trying to force you to eat something you don't want to.

5. You have the right to ask for what you want while accepting that asking doesn't always mean getting.

You can ask in a restaurant if they will give you a half portion for your main course. Maybe some won't oblige, but there is no harm in asking.

6. You have the right to be listened to and taken seriously.

Everyone's opinions should be respected, so if you have said you don't want to eat something, then of course you should be taken seriously. Maybe you have always eaten a takeaway every Friday night with the family, but now you'd rather not. If you have never stood up for yourself before, though, your friends and family may not be used to it. The more you do it, the more natural it will become.

7. You have the right to set your own priorities and state your own needs.

Figure out what your priorities are. If losing weight is one of them, then you need to stick to this rather than being swayed by other people's priorities. Always remember, your needs are just as important as anyone else's.

I think you will agree that these rules are good common sense and you would encourage family and friends to live by them, so why are you so different? Why don't you deserve the same respect?

Once you take on board what your basic rights are, it's really difficult to use them only when eating. You will hopefully notice that you start to abide by them in general life situations as well, not just at the dinner table.

In general, the aim of this weight loss plan is that it will become interwoven in your whole approach to life so that you are no longer just doing the techniques to lose weight, but you are doing them to improve your emotional well-being. They, therefore, become easier to carry on forever, rather than just until you reach a target weight. We have already discussed what happens when people stop their "fantastic" fad diet – obviously, the weight piles back on.

As well as the odd spike on your weight chart (as I said before, you cannot lose weight every week), there will come a time when your weight plateaus over several weeks. At this stage you have to decide if this is a healthy weight for you to stay at. If it is, you have done really well to reach it, and all you need to do is carry on as you are, consistently using all the techniques that have helped you to reach your goal. If, however, you feel you still want to lose a few more pounds, you might want to try increasing the amount of exercise you do and reduce the amount of calories you are taking in. A small change such as adding an extra fifteen or twenty minutes onto your usual exercise routine, or decreasing your calorie intake by around 200 calories per day (assuming you are not already at the minimum level of calorie intake), should make a difference over a couple of weeks so stick with it.

Checklist

1. Be realistic – it's okay to put on a few pounds during a holiday period.

2. It's easier than you think to carry on with these simple techniques during holidays to minimise weight gain.

3. Don't stop eating out and enjoying your food.

4. Deal with forceful feeders by becoming aware of the importance of your own goals and not giving in to other people's wishes all the time.

5. Remember these are lifelong changes. If you have found them helpful, why would you stop using them?

Chapter 11

Conclusion

It would be far too simplistic to say that losing weight alone has made me happy, as there are many factors that have contributed to my sense of overall wellbeing. However, maintaining a healthy weight is definitely one of those factors, because now it is simply one less thing that I have to worry about or feel bad about.

I love the feeling of being able to wear whatever I want to, without worrying if it will fit. For someone like me who adores clothes, this is a real benefit to losing weight. You need to find your driving factor, too. Your driving factor is that which is more important than everything else. Yes, I love food and eating out, but I love feeling good in my clothes even more. This, coupled with the knowledge that I don't actually have to give up all the food I love – I only need to eat mindfully and in moderation – is a win-win situation for me.

What is your driving factor? Is it to have more energy to play with your children? A sense of achievement in fulfilling a personal goal? Liking what you see when you look in the mirror? To lower your risk of diabetes? To wear that fantastic dress you bought that you've never been able to zip up? Think of your personal goals every day. They are the reason you are putting a little less on your plate, and walking a little further every day. The trade-off has to be worth it for you; it's your choice, but I know it was worth it for me.

I believe in leading by example, and I would not share my insights into losing weight if I didn't truly believe they worked. I know they work, because five years after losing weight, I am still maintaining it and have no intention of putting the weight back on again.

For many people, losing weight alone will not make them any happier, but unfortunately it's out with the scope of this book to deal with all the other problems in life. However, losing weight can be a great place to start, and making one successful change quite often leads onto lots of others. Achieving my ideal weight has also spurred me on to make other changes in my life. From supporting others through this weight loss plan, I have now decided to expand into personal styling and life coaching to encourage other people to make the best of themselves and achieve their goals, because life is too short to be stuck in a rut.

What you will find in this book are techniques that I have suggested to help you lose weight, but which will easily transfer to other situations to help you deal with them more effectively, too.

If your weight is your main issue in life and everything else is going pretty well, then I hope that by losing your excess weight you will find yourself even more content.

There are countless excuses for being overweight. Some people say they put on weight when they are in a relationship because they are comfortable and eating out more or have less time for exercise; others say they put on weight when their relationship is going badly and they are dissatisfied; yet other people claim to be overweight because they are unhappy that they are not in a relationship at all. You can see how easy it is to mould your current situation into being the reason for your weight gain. But by doing so, you are missing the point. You need to disentangle your eating habits from your life situation. Eating is not a solution to any other state, apart from hunger.

Perhaps you're thinking that this is easy for me to say but that it won't work for you. Although I have been through an intensive training course in Cognitive Behavioural Therapy, which obviously helped, the techniques that I use now are made for anyone to adopt and try out. I used to be extremely shy and would panic for weeks about having to give a presentation, yet now I regularly coach groups and have even delivered a workshop at Glasgow University.

I used to struggle to deal with cravings and would have no control over what I ate. Now I feel much more in control of what I eat, and therefore I feel more in control of my body.

I chose to make changes. I chose to use these techniques to make me feel better about myself – and you can choose to use them, too. Making excuses to not do so is only denying yourself the chance to be happy, so choose a different way today.

I didn't set out to lose as much weight as I did, but I found it so easy to stick to and the techniques so simple that I couldn't help but keep losing weight. I was aiming to lose 1.5 stones in the beginning, and I achieved this within three months.

Other diets may tease you with the promise that you can lose that amount of weight more quickly – and maybe you can. But I believe that the quicker you lose it, the harder it is to keep it off as you will most likely have had to make some drastic and uncomfortable changes in order to lose that much so quickly.

I was ecstatic when I reached the weight I thought I wanted to be, but because these lifestyle changes were now embedded in my life, I continued to lose weight – another stone, in fact – without feeling like I was trying to. This time of continuing weight loss covered the Christmas period and a holiday abroad with friends, so it proves that it is possible to lose weight while still enjoying life to the full. A weight loss plan should not impact on your life!

As I explained at the beginning of the book, you cannot lose weight every single week and I certainly didn't either, but the overall trend was a downward one and that is what you are aiming to achieve. After around six months, my weight continued to stay at the same level, give or take 2-3lbs. And as I had lost almost double what I had intended when I started out, I knew this was my natural weight so I am more than happy with it. It is now five years since reaching this weight and I have continued to stay within that parameter of 2-3lbs. Because I am still monitoring it, I always return to my target weight, rather than spiralling out of control as it might once have done when I was in denial.

I still wouldn't say that I am on a diet; all that is different is my attitude towards food. I like to use the example of "The French Paradox". A recent televised study on the world's best diets showed that France had the eighth best diet in the world in terms of health outcomes, such as heart disease, cholesterol levels, and life expectancy. Yet this seems contrary to the high fat diet they tend to indulge in. The French are world renowned for their cuisine and love of food, which includes cheese, pate, bread, red meat, red wine, pastries – all the things we are constantly warned against in this country. So why do they have such a good life expectancy and low rates of cardiovascular disease? I believe it's all in their attitude to food, which is exactly what this CBT approach is all about, too. Rather than a sense of deprivation and diet food, or "good" and "bad" food and seeing weight and food as a chore like calorie counting, avoiding meals out, etc, I believe the ideal mind-set to get into is that of the French.

The French culture celebrates food and the thought of grabbing a quick sandwich for lunch on the run would fill them with horror. Food in France is savoured and enjoyed, very much in line with the mindfulness principles of the CBT approach. They tend towards having three meals per day of good quality food, and rarely snack. This can be done easily and cheaply with proper meal planning. They have a little bit of what they fancy, similar to the wisdom of my grandmother's generation. A little bit does us no harm, it's the huge amounts we consume which is the problem. This links into the idea of portion control but not deprivation, and also not viewing food as "good" or "bad". In this way the French are very rational thinkers when it comes to food, rather than beating themselves up over enjoying a pain au chocolat or a delicious cheeseboard.

You will notice that I have not chosen the world's number one diet here (which was the Icelandic diet, in case you are interested), but the one which most closely shadows the principles of CBT and still maintains good health and weight outcomes. There are seven countries which are believed to have healthier diets than the French and I guess following the healthiest diet is the ideal. However, if we are to stick to realism – which, after all, is the basis of CBT – we could do a lot worse than adopt the French attitude to food. The fact that Scotland came in at a lowly number thirty-seven on the list of healthiest diets, compared to France at number eight, shows the huge gap between the two countries' eating habits.

Throughout the top ten of the world's best diets the points that stood out most to me were that these countries eat the least amount of processed food and stick closest to a traditional diet, rather than adopting the fast food culture that has endangered many developed nations. In general, meal times are enjoyed and food is really savoured. These points tend to be an important aspect of the country's culture and way of life.

I have deliberately avoided giving any suggestions as to what food you should be eating. That is because I am not a dietician. I do not have any specialist knowledge on what is good or bad for your health, other than the common sense information I have taken in like the rest of you. However, this study of the world's best diets does indicate that it's good common sense to opt for wholesome, unprocessed alternatives as often as possible, rather than processed, fast food, laden with chemicals and excess amounts of sugar and fat.

In our country, it can sometimes feel like food is seen as "the enemy" rather than something to be enjoyed. It is a quick fix to be dashed through at mealtimes but then relied upon to deal with all of life's' other problems. Food can only deal with hunger, not anything else!

Luckily for you, though, you have the ability to make choices, and you don't have to blindly follow the nation as a whole. It is too easy to blame other people or blame society for your weight gain, but that is very disempowering. If you feel like it is society or your genes' fault that you are overweight, then it is impossible to motivate yourself to change because you don't think it is your responsibility to do so.

If you can take full responsibility for what you eat, all of a sudden there is nowhere to hide and you become accountable for your weight. Denial and blame prevent us from dealing with the issue at hand. In a very small number of cases, of course, there is a medical reason why you may gain weight or find it a struggle to lose weight. That is why you should get checked out by your GP first of all to discount any underlying medical condition. This is an example of taking responsibility for yourself, because if you do find out you have a condition affecting your weight, you can then begin to be proactive in seeking expert advice to deal with it. Either way, the solution lies within ourselves, so grab it and start losing your weight now.

I hear many people say that losing weight is the easy bit but maintaining it is much harder. I think I may be in a strange minority, as I actually find starting out much harder, but once I have established a new routine then I find this quite easy to maintain. Either way, we all have hurdles to overcome when it comes to losing weight, but everything worthwhile in life has some challenges to deal with. The key is to keep focussed on how amazing you will feel once you have bounded over these hurdles.

I have never considered for a moment going back to my old habits as I feel so much better now than I ever did. I feel in control of my body, I feel proud that I have achieved a goal that I set for myself, and I feel fitter and more able to do whatever I want and wear whatever I want without being constrained by an out-of-shape body.

If I can do it, so can you. This time next year (or even next month), you will look back and be glad you gave it a try. Good Luck!

Bibliography

Beck, Judy (2007). *The Beck Diet Solution*

Burns, David (2000). *10 Days to Great Self Esteem*

Cannon, Geoffrey (2008). *Dieting Makes You Fat*

Frankl, Victor (1946). *Man's Search for Meaning*

Hamilton, David (2008). *How Your Mind Can Heal Your Body*

Hirschmann, Jane & Munter, Carol (1989). *Overcoming Overeating*

Roth, Geneen (1989). *Why Weight? A Guide to Ending Compulsive Eating*

SCOTACS Glasgow Gates Bill of Rights

http://www.mindtools.com/pages/article/newCDV_90.htm

http://psychology.about.com/od/personalitydevelopment/fl/What-Is-Locus-of-Control.htm

http://en.wikipedia.org/wiki/Locus_of_control

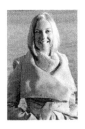

About the author

Having graduated from the University of Glasgow with an MA Honours Degree (Social Sciences) in 2006, Heather went on to train as a psychotherapist and holds a Diploma in Counselling and Groupwork - A CBT Approach. She spent several years assisting student therapists through their training as well as providing 1:1 therapy to a varied client group before deciding to specialise in weight loss after successfully losing 2 1/2 stone herself using cognitive behavioural methods. She has since run both weight loss groups and 1:1 sessions and more recently has facilitated psycho-educational workshops on the subject at the University of Glasgow.

I'd love to hear how you got on reading this book. If you have any comments or would like to enquire about attending my weight loss group or 1:1 programme please email me at

heather@keepitoff.me.uk

Learn more at

www.keepitoff.me.uk

Lightning Source UK Ltd.
Milton Keynes UK
UKOW06f0613110116

266156UK00001B/76/P